Because
It
Feels
Good

Because It Feels Good

A WOMAN'S GUIDE
TO SEXUAL PLEASURE
AND SATISFACTION

Debby Herbenick, PhD

RODALE

Notice

This book is intended as a reference volume only, not as a medical manual.
The information given here is designed to help you make informed decisions
about your health. It is not intended as a substitute for any treatment that may
have been prescribed by your doctor. If you suspect that you have a medical
problem, we urge you to seek competent medical help.

Sex and Values at Rodale

We believe that an active and healthy sex life, based on mutual consent and respect
between partners, is an important component of physical and mental well-being. We
also respect that sex is a private matter and that each person has a different opinion of
what sexual practices or levels of discourse are appropriate. Rodale is committed to
offering responsible, practical advice about sexual matters, supported by accredited
professionals and legitimate scientific research. Our goal—for sex and all other
topics—is to publish information that empowers people's lives.

© 2009 by Debby Herbenick, PhD, MPH

Rodale books may be purchased for business or promotional use or for special sales.
For information, please write to:
Special Markets Department, Rodale Inc., 733 Third Avenue, New York, NY 10017

Printed in the United States of America
Rodale Inc. makes every effort to use acid-free ♾, recycled paper ♺.

Book design by Susan P. Eugster
Illustrations are by Christopher M. Brown, Indiana University School of Medicine,
Office of Visual Media

Library of Congress Cataloging-in-Publication Data

Herbenick, Debby.
    Because it feels good : a woman's guide to sexual pleasure and satisfaction /
Debby Herbenick.
        p.   cm.
    Includes bibliographical references and index.
    ISBN-13: 978-1-60529-876-4 (hardcover)
    ISBN-10: 1-60529-876-X (hardcover)
    1. Sex instruction for women.   2. Sexual excitement.   I. Title.
HQ46.H45 2009
613.9'6082—dc22   2009006763

Distributed to the trade by Macmillan

2   4   6   8   10   9   7   5   3   1   hardcover

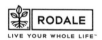

For my parents, who encouraged me
to laugh, to dance, and to love.

Whenever you are sincerely pleased you are nourished.
—Ralph Waldo Emerson

kisses are a better fate than wisdom.
—e.e. cummings

Contents

Reclaiming Pleasure

Learning How to Say No
Means More Yes, Yes, Yes!

Forget sex without love. Many women—whether they are in love, out of love, avoiding love, or hesitatingly dipping their toes into love—are having sex without *pleasure*. They might feel stuck in a rut, anxious that they aren't good enough lovers, focused entirely on their partner's desires rather than on their own, or resigned to thinking that adequate sex is as good as it gets. Others may be longing for affection but aren't sure how to reconnect with a partner who seems distant or disinterested. Still other women and men may feel like their sex lives, while not great, are decent enough, and the tips they've heard and techniques they've read about for having bigger, stronger orgasms or more exciting sex have ended up making sex feel too scripted. Rather than being blissfully absorbed in a rich experience of pleasure and intimacy, past attempts at learning new sex techniques have made them feel like they're following recipe instructions or the assembly manual for a piece of furniture.

If any of these scenarios sound familiar, you're not alone. Many people want to improve their experience of sexuality. Fortunately, you have the power—and here in this book, the information—to change your romantic or sexual life in a positive way and create pleasurable, sustainable sex (more on what that means later). Before we get in too deep, however, let's warm up with a little quiz.

POP QUIZ

1. In a 2007 study of college students, what was the number one reason that both women and men gave for having sex with another person?

> **a.** They felt attracted to the person
> **b.** They wanted to marry the person
> **c.** They wanted to become pregnant
> **d.** Because it seemed fun

2. In the past year, approximately what percentage of women and men likely had a period of several months during which they didn't find sex to be pleasurable?

> **a.** 10% of women and 1% of men
> **b.** 15% of women and 5% of men
> **c.** 23% of women and 8% of men
> **d.** 30% of women and 10% of men

3. Women who approach sex from a perspective of intimacy, calmness, or wanting to learn more about their partner are more likely to:

    a. Experience orgasm
    b. Masturbate
    c. Be single
    d. None of the above

4. Sexual satisfaction is most closely tied to:

    a. Penis size
    b. Relationship satisfaction
    c. Sex toy use
    d. Being single

Answers: 1) a; 2) c; 3) a; 4) b

How did you do? Did any of your answers surprise you? At the beginning of each chapter, I've included a quiz. The goal of this is to have you start thinking about various sex-related topics and what you'd like out of your sex life. This book, after all, is about celebrating the potential for sex to feel good—not just good as in toe-curling orgasms, but good as in you feel satisfied to the core of your being. It is also an invitation to explore how scientific information about sex can be used to enhance your experience of sexuality and to make intimacy more fun and fulfilling. That's true whether your sex life is shared with a partner, a vibrator, or a bit of each, and whether you are new to sex and relationships or well-seasoned in their ups and downs.

In subsequent chapters, we'll focus on specific topics

related to our bodies, sexual arousal, desire, orgasm, sex toys, positions, communication, and various tools that can help make feel-good sex achievable for you. First, however, we'll consider the differences between pleasurable and unpleasurable sex (beyond the obvious fact that one feels good and the other doesn't) and work on getting you more of the sex that you want and less of the sex you're less keen on. Specifically, after reading this chapter I hope that you will:

✳ Understand how women and men become caught in cycles of dread

✳ Be able to identify at least one strategy that you can use to prevent (or get out of) a cycle of dread

✳ Learn how to decline sex in a way that actually enhances your relationship

✳ Begin to pay more attention to the sensual nature of your sex life—the sights, sounds, scents, textures, and tastes

✳ Be able to articulate what you want your sex life to look and feel like

I wanted to write a book about the pleasures of sex because over the past few years, I've become concerned that many people have lost sight of how good sex can feel, inside and out. It seemed to me that sex had increasingly become just another thing on many people's to-do (or to-dread) lists. It seemed, too, that certain pressures had developed around sex. Some of these were new versions of old issues, like the pressure to perform (now intensified by a decade of performance-enhancing medications like Viagra) and the pressure to keep up sexually with the neighbors (highlighted in 2008 by the publication of

365 Nights: A Memoir of Intimacy, a book by a married woman who chronicled her year of daily sex with her husband[1]). When it seems like everyone else is having frequent and amazing sex—thanks in part to medication and exaggeration—many people begin to wonder whether their own sexual experiences are good enough, occur often enough, or are exciting enough.

SEX WITH (HEALTH) BENEFITS

Over the past few years, I've noticed another growing trend: the suggestion that people should have sex because it is "healthy." As a sex researcher at the Center for Sexual Health Promotion at Indiana University, Bloomington, and a sex educator at the Kinsey Institute, numerous newspaper, magazine, and online writers have interviewed me for articles about the "health benefits of having sex" or the "health-related reasons that people should have sex."

Collaborating with journalists is interesting work, particularly because they are a smart and curious bunch, and these stories were intended to help people improve their lives. Yet something about these "health benefit" articles began to frustrate me. Many of the articles seemed to highlight similar lines of research: namely, that having sex can reduce stress, lower blood pressure, boost immunity, relieve headaches, burn calories, reduce cancer risk, and encourage sound sleep. The implied advice was that women and men should have more sex more often—if not to save their relationships, then to save (or at least improve) their health.

The fact is, many of those benefits have been exaggerated or misrepresented. For example, while having sex can potentially reduce stress, it can also *increase* stress if the participant is worried about infection, pregnancy risk, emotional connection, or sexual performance. And while having sex burns some calories, it is rarely as effective an exercise as running, using the elliptical machine, or even taking a vigorous walk (unless you're having sex in a surprisingly athletic way!).

Don't get me wrong—as a sexual health and public health professional, it thrills me to no end when I read (or am interviewed for) positive articles about sex. Though it is important for women and men to understand the very real risks of having sex so that they can protect themselves physically and emotionally, our society spends so much time talking about the "bad" things that it's easy to forget that most of the sex we engage in is associated with positive, and often pleasurable, feelings or outcomes. When it comes to sex, I think we could all benefit from a more balanced perspective.

That said, and as much as I appreciate the fact that sex can improve health, I have to ask: Are health benefits primary *reasons* to have sex? The idea of living in a world in which people only have sex to burn calories does not appeal to me. From my perspective, having sex mainly to lower blood pressure is like eating a strawberry only because it is low in calories. Where is the joy in that? Call me a romantic, but toward the top of every person's list of "reasons to have sex," I would like to see the words "Because it feels good." Just as I eat a strawberry for its taste, its texture, and the way the juice dribbles down my chin when I bite into it, I'd hope we could embrace the sensual value of sex. I'm not suggesting that people can't ever have sex to relieve cramps or to help them fall asleep. People have sex for hundreds, probably thousands, of reasons, all of which are highly personal and valid. But most of the time, it should be about pleasure.

In August 2007, at the peak of the sex-for-health craze, I was happy to see the results of a study conducted by researchers from the University of Texas. Of the 237 reasons that college students cited for having sex, the third most common reason offered by women—and the second most common reason given by men—was "It feels good." ("Feeling attracted to the person" and "To experience physical pleasure" were the other top two reasons.) *Finally,* I thought. *Evidence that people don't just have sex to lower their blood pressure!* And yet, although the study got picked up by numerous media outlets, articles about the health benefits of sex continued to proliferate—and still do.

RECLAIMING PLEASURE

Aside from the fact that our society is in the midst of an overall health craze (consider the popularity of yoga, wheat grass, weight-loss reality shows, and smoking bans), I think that one of the reasons why "healthy sex" articles have become so popular is that many people are looking for reasons to feel good about sex in a world that often makes people feel bad about sex. Consider the numerous ways in which our culture makes people feel bad or uncomfortable about sex. Although most young children touch their genitals because they are curious, itchy, have diaper rash, or think it feels good, some parents and caregivers still warn children not to touch "down there," implying that doing so is "dirty" or "bad." Depending on the family, culture, or religion in which a child is raised, there may be other forms of guilt, shame, or embarrassment that come to be associated with sex. As kids grow up, they may be warned about the risks and dangers of sex, or they may get messages (both verbal and nonverbal) about a double standard: Young women who are sexual with others are sluts or have low self-esteem, whereas young men who are sexual with others are confident and popular (or at least "just being guys"). As young women and men begin having sex, they may struggle with how to transform an act that has been described as bad, dangerous, or shameful into an expression of love, intimacy, or joy. They may also worry endlessly about their ability to have strong erections, achieve orgasm easily, last long enough, or twist their bodies into practically acrobatic positions.

Therein lies a paradox. Although people commonly have sex for reasons related to pleasure, we know that sex doesn't always feel good. In fact, one nationally representative study of women and men reported that a full 23 percent of women and 8 percent of men said that during the previous year they had gone at least several months without feeling that their experience of sex was pleasurable. That's a lot of people to be feeling "blah" or even bad about sex *within just one year!* You can imagine how many more people have found sex to be unpleasurable at some other point in their lives—probably most of us.

We also know that even when sex *does* feel good, pleasure isn't the one and only reason that people seek it out. That 2007 study of college students doesn't represent the whole picture. As you likely know, although attraction, pleasure, and raging hormones may be the primary reasons why young adults or those in new relationships have sex, over time those reasons change. With an average age of 19, few (if any) participants in that study had experienced how sexual attitudes can alter in response to life-changing events like pregnancy, hysterectomy, aging, illness, parenthood, menopause, or simply feeling burned out after years or decades of working at a full-time job. At different times in people's lives or relationships, there will

●

be different motivations to have sex. For many couples, starting a family is a major reason to have sex. While making a baby can feel exciting and arousing, sometimes it can also feel worrisome, stressful, or sad (particularly if pregnancy doesn't happen as easily as expected or at all).

Other women and men look around one day and realize that a good chunk of the sex they've had over the previous month or year was more about making their partner—not themselves—feel good. Has that ever happened to you or a friend? Maybe you noticed that sometimes you had sex because you worried that if you didn't, you might disappoint your partner, or he or she might leave you for someone with a higher sex drive. Or you hoped that your partner would stop nagging if you gave in. (Or the opposite might be true—you wished you didn't have to nag your partner to have sex with you.) Then again, maybe you pulled your partner into the bedroom or grabbed a vibrator from the nightstand simply to relieve tension, de-stress, or fall asleep more easily. You may have even found yourself having sex with someone new because you felt so utterly betrayed, rejected, or hurt by someone you love that you sought revenge—or solace—in another person's arms. All of these are reasons that people give for having sex, but not all of them are paths to "feel good" sex. And if you're reading this book, then it is probably a safe assumption that the kind of sex you want—at least more of the time—is sex that feels pleasurable, enjoyable, satisfying, and maybe even sends tingles up and down your spine.

SUSTAINABLE SEX

Most people—no matter how much emotional satisfaction or intellectual stimulation their relationships provide—have a

Sex and Your Senses

Many people find that they can enhance their sexual experiences by paying attention to the sensual nature of their encounters. Read through the examples below and think about the things you notice while having sex. See if you can add one or two of your own sensual experiences to each of these categories, and indulge in noticing and enjoying them the next time you have sex (privately or with a partner).

SIGHT

Bodies; using candlelight or a dimmer switch to change how the light shines on your bodies; wearing lingerie; the look of your own or your partner's body in the shower, wrapped in a bath towel, in a swimsuit, or dressed up to go out; the freckles or wrinkles on your partner's skin; the way that your partner smiles or looks at you with love or lust.

SOUND

The sound of your partner's voice; moans and sighs; changes in breathing patterns during sexual excitement; special pet names that your partner has for you; the sound of your vibrator at different speeds; whispered words; laughing at funny moments during sex.

SCENT

Body scents; how body scents change after sex; scented candles or massage products; perfume or cologne; bubble bath; how bodies smell right out of the shower, after working out, or when you're hugging versus making love.

TOUCH/FEEL

The feel of your naked bodies pressed against each other; hair-covered body parts; hairless body parts; soft curves; sharp angles; using a feather to tease one another; different types of touch (like soft, hard, quick, slow, tongue, hands, wet, dry, cold, warm).

TASTE

Kissing or licking your partner's body; flavored lubricant or edible body dust; body fluids; using food (like whipped cream or chocolate) as a playful part of sex; how kisses taste different after brushing teeth, eating certain foods, or first thing in the morning.

need to feel sexually desirable or gratified. It is okay to want that, and it is wise to seek out information about improving your experience of sex if that feels important to you or to your relationship.

My primary goal in writing this book is to help you claim a larger proportion of your sexual experiences as sex that feels good—the kind of sex that makes you glad that you left the dirty dishes in the sink and opted for refuge in your bedroom. The sex that I am referring to is not necessarily "mind-blowing sex," a term sometimes used among friends and in women's magazines, though at times it might feel that way. My term for the kind of sexual experience I want you to be able to achieve for yourself is "yummy sex"—the kind that makes you smile and blush even hours after you've had it. In addition to being blush-worthy, yummy sex is also sustainable over your lifetime—it's not just reserved for the young or newly coupled. It is sex that feels sensual and evocative, that is flexible and responsive to the ebbs and flows of aging, relationships, and life changes.

CYCLES OF DREAD

In our journey toward achieving satisfying, sustainable sex, let's be clear that no matter how much you learn about sex or get in touch with your sensuality, sex won't always feel fantastic—or even good. Sometimes sex—in spite of our best knowledge, intentions, and emotions—doesn't feel the way we'd hoped, planned, or expected. Occasionally our bodies don't cooperate, the kids walk in, the phone rings in the middle of the night, the batteries die, our partners disappoint us, or we disappoint ourselves. In fact, research suggests that when happily committed couples have sex, although it feels good the vast majority of the time, about 5 to 15 percent of their experiences were described as unsatisfying or problematic (and another 15 to 20 percent were described as "fair," rather than good). Other times, we don't necessarily desire sex. You may have had the experience of feeling tired, overworked, sick, mad, confused about your relationship, or just not in the mood. And yet you may have had sex not because you wanted to, but because you felt that—for some reason—you *should* have sex.

On the surface, this might seem harmless. After all, isn't having sex with your partner when he or she wants to the nice thing to do, even if you'd rather curl up in bed with a book? An occasional, altruistic "gift" to your partner is unlikely to cause any harm. In fact, many women and men find that once they start with foreplay, they become aroused, and they soon find that they are happy that they decided to have sex. Sound familiar? It's similar to how some people feel when they make themselves go to the gym or go for a walk. Even if they didn't feel like it at first, once people get their bodies going, their minds sometimes follow.

However, some women find themselves giving in and having sex that they don't want and may feel too tired for, only to find that over time it creates what I call a "cycle of dread." When this happens, they begin to dread not only sex, but also any sign of affection from their partner. A simple kiss, hug, pat on the butt, or back rub can trigger resistance because they fear it may possibly lead to sex. They learn to dread the potential for sex because sex itself, or the way the sexual interaction makes them feel, has become unpleasurable.

When, over a period of time, you repeatedly have sex that doesn't feel good (emotionally or physically) and that you don't really want, you may begin to reject offers of affection. When your partner tries to give you a kiss, you turn your head and offer a cheek, thinking, "I'd better not kiss back or he'll think I want to have sex." As the cycle continues, he may stop kissing and hugging you (for fear of being rejected), which causes you to stop feeling desirable, and then sex—if it happens at all— probably doesn't feel very good, intimate, or pleasurable. He may be thinking you don't desire him (since you often dread and recoil from kisses), and you may be thinking he doesn't desire you, either (since he has initiated affection less and less often). It is difficult to lose yourself in passionate abandon when you don't want to be naked and vulnerable in bed with another person, when you feel alone in a relationship, or when you question why your partner stopped kissing you the way he or she used to. Often this repeated cycle of dread and pleasure- less sex can lead to bigger problems with sexual interest, desire, arousal, or orgasm—all of which we will tackle together in the chapters to come. First, however, let's consider ways to avoid getting caught in a cycle of dread, as well as how to get out of one and bring pleasure back.

The Roots of Dread

Cycles of dread can be caused, or made worse, by having sex over and over again when you don't want it, thus setting yourself up for sex that doesn't feel good. Now remember: There is nothing wrong (and there is plenty that's right) with occasion- ally having sex even if you're not in the mood at first. That said, there are times when both women and men just don't want to have sex—and that's okay. No one should be made to feel like they should have sex if the fact is that they don't want it. It's normal to feel "blah" about sex at times. If you're exhausted or weary, you may be better off getting some rest. If you're feeling distant from or upset with your partner, you may both benefit

What Kind of Sex Do You Want to Have?

Like any journey, the path to pleasurable sex is made easier if you have an idea of where you'd like to go. Read through this list and consider which words or phrases best describe how you would like sex to feel. You can choose as many as you would like, as sex feels different at different times. You may even find that you want intercourse to feel one way and self-pleasuring (masturbation) to feel another. If it's easier, place letters or symbols by words to denote different things—for example, an "m" for words that describe how you want your masturbation to be or an "i" for how you'd like intercourse to feel.

Pleasing	Overwhelming	Hard	Wet
In control	Soft	Orgasmic	Pleasurable
Happy	Dry	Gentle	Funny
Enrapturing	Seductive	Sensible	Vigorous
Meaningful	Safe	Fun	Satisfying
Rough	Loving	Trusting	Easy
Casual	Challenging	Spiritual	Interesting
Curious	Lustful	Exciting	Long-lasting
Enthusiastic	Quick	Meditative	Energetic
Relaxing	Slow	Ecstatic	Erotic
Beautiful	Sexy	Euphoric	Sassy
Emotional	Cheeky	Powerful	Wild
Tender	Secure	Restrained	Connecting
Intimate	Tense	Imaginative	Close
Comfortable	Inspiring	Reassuring	Secretive
Bonding	Sneaky	Playful	Natural
Light-hearted	Deep	Serious	Flirtatious

What other words come to mind? How else would you like to experience sex? Keep these ideas in mind as we move forward and work on creating sexual experiences that feel right (or desirable) to you.

from talking it out rather than having sex that makes you feel lonely. In my opinion, and given that our culture is obsessed with having enormous amounts of sex, we don't acknowledge often enough that not only is it okay to not always want sex, but that it also makes perfect sense that we don't want sex all of the time. I'd rather have good quality than high quantity anyway, wouldn't you?

You may have heard the widely quoted statistic that 43 percent of women have some kind of sexual dysfunction—a number that has made many women question their own sex lives. But that figure is highly controversial, and it doesn't necessarily present an accurate picture. What the research does show is that about 43 percent of women have experienced stretches of time during which they've had problems like low desire or interest and difficulty achieving an orgasm. But not one of these common issues necessarily qualifies as a "dysfunction." In fact, only about 24 percent of those women reported to actually *feel bothered* by these sexual issues (which is closer to the definition of a "dysfunction"). In other words, women aren't as sexually dysfunctional as some news reports or pharmaceutical companies might lead you to believe. That's not to say that 24 percent of women feeling bothered by sexual problems is a low number—in fact, I think it screams the need for quality sex education and resources.

Preventing Dread: Learning to Say No

In learning to attract yummy sex, it is important for women and men to develop the skills to choose the sex that they want and take rain checks on the rest. And yet, that's not a skill that many of us have ever learned. If you think about it, the only two types of sex that most people have ever been taught to say "no" to are

●

underage, teenage sex ("If he tries anything, just tell him no"), and nonconsensual sex, in the context of rape ("No means no"). And yet the vast majority of times in our lives that we say no to sex do not involve either of those situations. Most of the time, the type of sex that we want to say no to is sex with someone we love or care deeply about. This can feel daunting, as it can be difficult to reject—and thus risk hurting or offending—someone we're crazy for.

We're never really given any guidance on how to say no to sex that we just aren't in the mood for—unless, of course, you count learning from the old "Not tonight, dear; I have a headache" joke. And sadly, the root of that joke is a person feigning illness to avoid sex. Where, then, do we learn how to decline sex in an honest, open way that clearly communicates our feelings to our partner? To say no without making one's partner feel rejected or hurt? Unsure of how to decline sex gently, many people just give in, which can make sex feel like a duty, an obligation, or something to dread.

How odd, you might be thinking, to begin a book about having sex that feels good by discussing how to decline sex that doesn't feel good. And yet it seems to me, based on my work with individuals and couples, that until we learn (and practice) how to decline sex that we *don't* want, it is difficult to fully embrace—and create more opportunities for—the sex that we crave. In this way, learning to say no is an important first step toward learning to say yes more often to sex that we *do* want: the blush-worthy kind.

Not Tonight, Dear, I'm . . .

In spite of the stereotype that it is mainly women who don't feel like having sex, men sometimes don't feel like it either. We probably see, read about, or watch women rejecting sex more often because it is culturally acceptable. Men are generally taught to be the initiators of sex—and if you're a guy who often initiates sex, then chances are that at least some of the time you'll be rejected. (As the old saying goes, whether it's with jobs or with dating, "If you're not getting rejections, you're not trying hard enough.") This myth that men are always "ready and willing" can create numerous complications for couples, from erection problems (which can occur when a man has sex because he feels as though he "should") to relationship problems (a woman may worry that if her boyfriend or husband turns down an opportunity for sex, he may have lost interest or he may be gay).

There are a lot of reasons why people sometimes aren't in the mood for sex, either privately or with a partner. Some common ones include:

* Stress

* Fatigue

* Boredom

* Health problems

* Hormonal changes

* Relationship problems

* Grief

* Concerns about risks (such as pregnancy, infection, or feeling emotionally hurt)

* Anxiety

* Feeling alone or misunderstood

* Low desire

* Medication side effects

All of these are valid reasons to not feel up to having sex or self-pleasuring, particularly given the fact that sex often requires both emotional and physical energy. However, just because these are valid reasons doesn't mean that people know how to express them effectively to a partner. We often make up reasons why we don't feel like having sex (the "I have a head-ache" strategy) or are vague ("I just don't feel like it"), rather than digging in, telling the truth, and clearly communicating with our partners. But your partner knows you too well to buy these lines, and the result is often heartbreaking. He or she may begin to question what you are hiding, what is behind the "no." When people's sexual advances are rejected, they may begin asking themselves any of the following questions:

✳ Does my partner still love me?

✳ Does my partner find me unattractive?

✳ Is my partner cheating on me?

✳ Have I done or said something wrong?

✳ Is this the beginning of the end of our sex life?

✳ Are we becoming one of those couples who never has sex?

✳ Is my partner mad at me?

But there is another option—you can say no to sex in a way that is both clear and careful of your partner's feelings. It's easier to do so if you:

✳ Are aware of the true reason you don't want to have sex

✳ Can communicate that reason to your partner

✳ Try to reassure your partner of his or her worth and attractiveness to you

✳ Suggest another way of being close, intimate, or sexual

●

FACT: *How you approach sex can shape how you experience it.*

Although orgasm isn't everything, it is an important part of sexual pleasure for many women and men. In a 2003 study,[2] women who found it difficult to orgasm were more likely to experience sex in ways that were related to guilt, shame, stress, anxiety, embarrassment, withdrawal, detachment, or concerns about being used. On the other hand, women who found it easier to orgasm were more likely to have experienced intercourse as related to love, intimacy, calmness, relief, or as a way to learn about oneself or one's partner. When you think of sex, what are the first feelings that come to mind? Are they related to delight or dread? Stress or relaxation? Try to use positive self-talk in ways that promote pleasure and connection.

MYTH: *Relationship satisfaction has little to do with sexual satisfaction.*

So much for the fiery couple who thrives on passionate, angry sex as a way to get over their numerous, angry fights. It's not that those couples don't exist—they do—but they're the minority. More often than not, sexual satisfaction is easier to come by when couples feel close, connected, understood, in love, happy with where they're at and where they're going, and equal in important ways.

Here are some examples.

"Considering how hot you look right now, I would love to, but I am absolutely exhausted from chasing the kids around today. Can I take a rain check for another night?"

"I'm completely attracted to you, but I'd like to get to know you better before we take it any further. I'd love to go out with you again."

"You know how much I love—and totally want—you, but my vagina still hurts for some reason. I'm going back to the doctor next week to see what's up . . . in the meantime, can we maybe try something other than intercourse, like making out or oral sex?"

"You have no idea how appealing that sounds, but I'm feeling really stressed and distracted about work, and I'm not sure I'll be up to par tonight. What would you think about masturbating while I watch?"

"For all our ups and downs, you're still my favorite person in the universe, and I love having sex with you. But I have to tell you: I'm still a little angry about what happened earlier today, and I'm not feeling in the right frame of mind for sex. Can we talk about it so I can figure it out in my head and get over it? Our relationship—and our sex life—is too important to me to let this come between us."

There's no getting around it—each of these rejections is still a rejection. That's life: Not everyone will always want to have sex when you do, and you will not always want to have sex when your partner does. Certainly we can learn to say no (or to hear no from our partner) without it signaling the end of love, lust, or our relationship.

The power of each of the above examples lies in the fact that the person saying no to sex also says something that validates their partner or their relationship, expresses a clear reason for saying no, and indicates that an effort is being made to enhance the relationship. This combination makes the "no" a rejection of sex at that very moment, rather than a rejection of the person, the relationship, or future opportunities to have sex. After all, relationship satisfaction is one of the most important elements to sexual satisfaction, so it's important to keep your connection alive.

Consider alternatives to sex that can help you feel close to your partner or indicate that you're still interested in being sexual or intimate in other ways. Study after study shows that masturbation, for example, is commonly enjoyed by both women and men who are in happy, committed, satisfying relationships—it is far from being only a "partner substitute." If you don't feel like having intercourse, perhaps you can watch each other masturbate or kiss your partner while he or she self-pleasures. Erotic touching, sensual massage, taking a shared bath, or rubbing each other's feet while sitting close together on the sofa are all possibilities, too.

Learning and practicing how to decline sex can take time, and it certainly helps if you have a partner who listens to what you say (and really hears it) and who is secure and confident enough with themselves and with your relationship to take a "no" in stride. Sometimes couples who have been together for a long time are used to their relationship routine, and change doesn't always feel good at first. It can feel scary and disruptive to suggest doing things a new way. If you find that negotiating when to have (or not have) sex is difficult for you or your partner, you might find it helpful to meet with a sex therapist or counselor. (See Resources on page 234 for more information.) If your partner is reluctant to attend therapy with you, try appealing to his helpful side. Let him know that sometimes you find it difficult to talk through relationship or sexuality issues, and you need his help. Suggest that you'd like to meet with a therapist not because things are bad, but because you value your relationship (and your sex life) and think that a sex therapist may have a lot to offer. By emphasizing his importance in your life, you may find that he will be open to the idea of professional guidance.

GOOD-BYE DREAD, HELLO PLEASURE!

If you're not currently stuck in a cycle of dread, the following exercises can help you to *prevent* dread. And if you have been dreading sex lately, try these ideas on for size and see if they can help create a cycle of desire. (In Chapter 3, we'll talk a lot more about enhancing desire.)

* **Practice gratitude.** Sometimes sex-dreaders find that they focus so much on the negative that they forget the positive. Research has shown that people can improve their relationships when they focus on good things about their partners and express appreciation. Every day, try to identify at least one thing for which you are grateful about your partner (he apologizes when he's wrong, kisses you when you come home) and one thing for which you are grateful about your relationship (you feel respected, admired, loved).

* **Nix the negative self-talk.** Human beings are storytellers. Most of our stories are ones that we tell ourselves. Notice what you say to yourself in relation to your partner. If he or she tries to have sex with you, do you find yourself making up a bad story in your head, such as, "He doesn't care about me or how my day was, he just wants to have sex"? If so, no wonder it's difficult to feel receptive to him! Try to stop the negative story and reframe it as, "He's so attracted to me, and loves me so deeply, that he can't keep his hands to himself." It's a much different

story, with a warmer feeling—and it's all just a matter of reframing your perspective.

✳ **Be open to change.** If you've been upset with your partner and find yourself thinking "he always does that" or "he'll never be who I want," then you may not be giving him the chance to change or yourself a chance to notice the progress he's made. Keeping score can take an emotional toll on both of you. Try to notice and encourage small steps in the right direction. Change takes time, and it benefits from positive reinforcement, rather than criticism or skepticism.

✳ **Embrace sensual pleasures.** How might you experience pleasure with your partner in ways that don't involve sex? Could you be more affectionate with kisses, hugs, or pats on the back? If he or she truly does spring into sex every time you offer affection, saying (gently, and with a smile) that "sometimes I just want to kiss" is one way to be clear about your intentions.

You don't have to use each of these strategies in order to inspire change in your relationship. Just try one or two as a start—and really devote yourself to it—to see what works for you.

HOMEWORK
Discover What Makes You Feel Good

Just as it's important to practice saying no to sex that we don't want, it is also important to become aware of what we *do* like and want so that we can say yes to things that intrigue us. Often, women and men I've worked with have found it easy (and fun) to practice this skill in both sexual and nonsexual situations. Here are some exercises you can try as you learn to identify your likes.

1. Go to the grocery store and rather than buying the usual foods, buy at least one food item that you think would feel really tasty in your mouth. Not your partner's or your child's mouth, but *your* mouth.

2. When it comes to television, watch at least one show that only *you* want to watch—and feel free to go into another room if a show comes on that you really don't want to see. You can always read, take a bath, go on a walk, or call a friend from another room in your home.

3. Look at your schedule. Which activities do you really enjoy? Which ones have you agreed to because you felt like you should, or because other people would be happy if you did?

4. Think about how you like to look, act, dress, or wear your hair. What's keeping you from that image? Is it a fear that women your age shouldn't have long hair or wear short skirts? Where are the boundaries between what you want and what you're uncomfortable having?

5. Spend some time figuring out what makes you feel sexy. Is there a certain shirt, dress, nightgown, or pair of pants that makes you feel desirable? What would you like to see your partner wear, as a turn-on?

6. Determine what types of foreplay or sex play are most arousing to you. What mix of sex would be most ideal to you—intercourse here and there, with occasional evenings of making out like you did as a teenager? Mutual masturbation? Watching each other play with sex toys?

7. Consider your kissing. Are there types of kissing that you miss or haven't done in a while? Would you like to be kissed gently on the forehead, on the lips with more tongue, or softly on your inner thighs?

I am not suggesting that you become selfish, but it's important to achieve a balance that will help you figure out what you like, as well as what you don't like. Give yourself permission to like things that you may not have liked or even considered in the past. We all change, and it is normal that your likes and dislikes may change from time to time. I've heard women say that they would love to pull their partner closer and tear his clothes off, but they worry about appearing too aggressive or "unfeminine." Similarly, many men I've spoken with have felt trapped by a cultural idea that men shouldn't want to cuddle after (or instead of) sex. If you can recognize what you want, as well as the artificial limits that you've placed on yourself, you can break through those boundaries and seek the pleasure, excitement, and satisfaction that you're capable of.

The steps we've taken so far can help move you in the direction of reclaiming sexual pleasure for yourself and your partner (if you have one). Learning to focus on pleasure and to decide that it's okay to have sex because it feels good, rather than to burn calories or to make someone else happy, form the foundation for the rest of this book. After all, if you don't feel that you deserve pleasurable sex—or if you are stuck thinking about it in very planned, artificial ways—it will be difficult to get excited about it. And this book is about helping you open up to the excitement, intimacy, and satisfaction you deserve.

Vulvas, Vaginas, and G-Spots, Oh My!

A Brief Anatomy Lesson

I wasn't born knowing everything about sex, nor do I know everything about it now. In fact, it wasn't until I was in my early twenties—and working as a research assistant at the Kinsey Institute—that I knew precisely what a vulva was. Sure, I had seen my vulva, but I had always thought that everything "down there" was called a vagina. I wasn't familiar with the word "vulva," nor did I know about all of its parts, except perhaps for the clitoris. Fast forward: It is the fall of 2007, and I've been asked to appear on *The Tyra Banks Show* to teach women about vulvas and vaginas with my Wondrous Vulva Puppet. Somehow, in less than a decade, I had gone from knowing nothing about the vulva to being an expert on a talk show episode devoted entirely to the vulva and vagina and called "What's up down there?"

When I arrived at the taping, I was asked to keep my vulva puppet in the green room and not take it out in the hallway or bring it into the hair and makeup room. I didn't understand why it was such a big deal, but I later learned that Barack Obama was in his own green room down the hall. The producers feared that the then presidential hopeful might accidentally come into contact with my anatomical puppet.

So much drama over a little vulva puppet! But the fact is that vulvas and vaginas make some people very uncomfortable. Talking about them used to make *me* feel uncomfortable. After all, most of us have been raised in a culture that supports the idea that women's genitals are dirty and need to be "cleaned up" with feminine hygiene products (not true!). Fortunately, as adults, we can learn more accurate information about our bodies, our sex lives, and our health that helps us to feel less squeamish and enables us to have more pleasurable sex. I don't expect you to adore these body parts like I do (though after reading this chapter, you might!), but I do want you to learn more about your vagina and vulva. An accurate understanding of your own anatomy is a vital part of embracing sexual pleasure and taking care of your sexual and reproductive health. And for those of you who are hoping to increase your arousal or more easily achieve orgasm, this knowledge is more important than you may realize. Stick with me.

Let's start with a quiz.

POP QUIZ

1. On average, the vagina is about:

    a. 3 to 4 inches long

    b. 5 to 6 inches long

    c. 7 to 8 inches long

    d. It depends on whether a woman is sexually aroused

2. The word "vulva" refers to a woman's:

    a. External genitals (her mons, clitoris, labia, and so on)

    b. Birth canal

    c. G-spot

    d. Vagina

3. The G-spot is:

    a. An area on the back wall of the vagina that, when stimulated, some but not all women find pleasurable

    b. Another term for the clitoris

    c. An area on the front wall of the vagina that, when stimulated, some but not all women find pleasurable

    d. An easily orgasmic spot for most women

4. On average, at what angle does the vagina rest?

    a. 90°

    b. 130°

    c. 160°

    d. It depends on a woman's arousal levels, hormone levels, and age

5. The most sensitive, nerve-rich part of a woman's genitals is her:

    a. Vagina

    b. Glans clitoris

    c. Labia minora

    d. G-spot

Answers: 1) d; 2) a; 3) c; 4) d; 5) b

Before I began studying sex, I would probably have answered only one of these five questions correctly, so don't worry if you missed a few. Nobody is keeping score and, as it turns out, there are no medals or awards for vulvovaginal knowledge or expertise. However, after you've read this chapter, I think you'll be surprised by how much you've learned about the parts you've lived with your entire life but never really knew. (Kind of like that anonymous neighbor you smile and wave at as you walk to your car each day.) You're about to get to know your vulva and vagina a whole lot better.

Even scientists and gynecologists have a lot to learn about our most private of parts. Thanks to tireless advocacy by women's groups and sexual health organizations, more researchers are studying women's genitals to better understand vaginal size, lubrication, pain during intercourse, orgasm, sexual arousal, and more. And every bit of this knowledge matters.

A lot of exciting research has been conducted on vaginas and vulvas over the last decade. It's shocking to me that much of this new information hasn't made it into mainstream media like magazines or sexual health books. The full size of the clitoris was only "discovered" and written about by scientists in the late 1990s, and many anatomy textbooks I've seen *still* don't include accurate diagrams of it. How are doctors and nurses supposed to learn about the clitoris if their textbooks aren't up to date?

I think you deserve access to the most accurate information possible about your body, especially since much of this knowledge can have an impact on your experience of sexual pleasure. It's important to understand the science behind common issues like why sex may feel less comfortable with age or after a hysterectomy so that you can learn how to continue experiencing sexuality with immense pleasure.

Even though all of us essentially come "from" the vagina, we somehow learn at a very early age not to talk about the vagina and vulva, as if they were dirty or unclean or anything but awe-inspiring. If you think that this sounds like crazy talk—that vaginas and vulvas are not awe-inspiring—please read this chapter twice. I won't try to convert you to vagina worship, but I do want to encourage you to think about these issues. For example, why are so many women and men embarrassed about their genitals? And how is it that so many of us women know so little about our own bodies?

My research suggests[1] that how we feel about our genitals matters, as women, to our gynecological and sexual health. Women who feel good about their vaginas and vulvas tend to be more likely to have an annual gynecological exam, to enjoy receiving oral sex, and to find it easy to orgasm. My research has also indicated that men actually have a more positive view of women's genitals than we women do. While I'm glad that they love our lady parts, isn't it about time we respected our bodies enough to understand and appreciate our genitals, too?

My goal is for you to learn enough about your body in this chapter that you can begin to feel more comfortable:

❋ Performing a monthly vulvar self-examination

❋ Exploring your own genitals to learn what feels pleasurable to you

❋ Asking your healthcare provider about any genital-related concerns you might have (such as questions about vaginal itch, odor, or pain during intercourse)

❋ Talking to your sexual partner about your body, what feels good to you, and what types of touching or stimulation you most enjoy and find pleasurable (as well as what you don't enjoy or don't find pleasurable)

✹ Teaching your daughter/sister/niece about her body and how to take care of it

✹ Encouraging your mother to take care of her gynecological health by performing vulvar self-examinations and going to her annual gyn exam

THE VULVA

When I teach college-level human sexuality classes, I show a huge PowerPoint slide of a Volvo with a big heading that says "A vulva is not a car." It may seem silly, but in my experience, both women and men are rarely familiar with the word "vulva." I explain that just as the word "face" refers to body parts like the forehead, cheeks, nose, and chin, the word "vulva" refers to the external parts of a woman's genitals, including the mons pubis, clitoral hood, glans clitoris, labia majora, labia minora, and vaginal entrance. In one study that my mentor and colleague Stephanie Sanders, PhD, and I conducted at the Kinsey Institute in 2002, we found that fewer than 20 percent of college-educated women could accurately describe what a vulva is. While it may not be a word that you hear or use very often, I want you to know what it means. Why? Because if you need to talk to your partner or healthcare provider about something involving your vulva (telling a partner where you want to be touched, describing discomfort to your doctor), you should be able to clearly communicate what you mean. If you say that your "vagina" hurts, your doctor will examine the inside of you. But if you say that your "vulva" hurts, your doctor will be able to understand and treat the parts that are causing you pain.

Later on I'll ask you to take out a mirror and find these parts on your own body. But for now, I just want you to take a few minutes to learn about them. As we move on through the book, we'll refer back to these parts and discuss how they relate to our capacity for pleasure, sensation, and intimacy. The diagram below will help you understand where each part is located.

Keep in mind that this is just a diagram used to illustrate where each part is. In reality, our vulvas all look somewhat different from each other. Some women have larger labia majora or labia minora, and other women have very tiny labia.

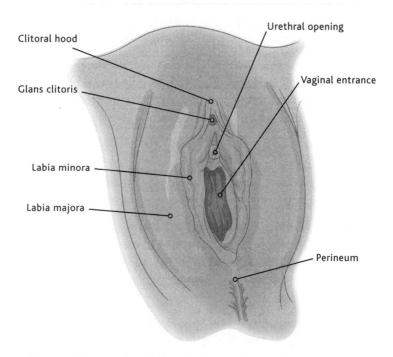

The parts of a woman's vulva (external genitals)

The glans clitoris (the part of the clitoris that you can see) varies in size, too, as can the coloration of each part.

The **mons pubis** is the triangular area of a woman's genitals that you can see when you stand in front of a mirror. Most girls begin to grow pubic hair on the mons pubis during puberty. The amount and thickness of pubic hair varies from sparse and thin to quite thick or bushy. This area is sometimes just called "the mons." It is also known as the Mound of Venus (remember Venus, the goddess of love?), which I think is a pretty good reminder of the sexy things that can take place around the vulva. Whether privately or with a partner, many women find that it feels pleasurable to stroke their mons or to gently tug on their pubic hair, stimulating the sensitive skin and nerve endings in this area.

If you sit on your bed with your legs spread apart and hold a mirror, you will see the more private parts of your vulva. These parts cannot usually be seen when you are naked in the locker room. They are typically only seen by you, your sexual partner, and your healthcare provider, though some girls or women have shown their vulvas to their very close friends in an effort to compare parts and get a sense of what is normal.

The **clitoral hood** is a fold of skin that protects the **glans clitoris**, which is tightly packed with nerve endings and consequently is often very sensitive to touch. When women talk about enjoying stimulation of "the clitoris" or "the clit," they often mean the glans clitoris, though they don't always know where it is located. In our study, fewer than 60 percent of women were able to correctly identify on a diagram where the clitoris was located. Considering that the clitoris is a power-house of sensation and pleasure, it would be good to know where to find it, either for private pleasuring or to show your

•

partner how you like to be touched. More than any other part of the vulva, the clitoris is packed with nerve endings and thus sensation. In fact, it has no other biological function than to experience sensation and hopefully promote pleasure. You don't pee from it. You don't make babies with it. And it doesn't have anything to do with your period. Typically you should be able to see about ¼ to ½ inch of the clitoris. However, as was described in 1998 by Australian researcher Helen O'Connell, MD, of the University of Melbourne, the clitoris is actually considerably bigger than that. It stretches back at an angle into the body in two branches of erectile tissue called **crura,** which measure about 3 or 3½ inches each.

Below the clitoris is the **urethral opening** through which women urinate. This is often much easier to see on diagrams than it is in real life when you're looking at your own body. The two reasons I think it's important to check out this part are 1) to understand that women do not pee from their vaginas (a popular misconception), and 2) because when you see how close the urethra is to the vagina, you can understand how vaginal discharge or sexual fluids (such as vaginal lubrication, store-bought lubricant, or ejaculate from a partner) can easily get inside the urethra and contribute to a urinary tract infection (UTI). This is why some women who are particularly prone to UTIs are often advised to drink lots of fluids and urinate after self-pleasuring or partner play. Flushing out any "foreign" substances or irritants from the body may help reduce the risk of developing a UTI.

Framing the vulva are the **labia majora**—a part of the vulva that fewer than one-third of women in our study could identify—sometimes referred to as the outer vaginal lips. ("Labia" is Latin for "lips.") There is typically some amount of hair on the outside of each labium (the singular of labia is "labium"). The **labia minora** (inner lips) are hairless and may be sensitive to touch. The labia minora vary widely from woman to woman. Some hang down only a ¼ or ⅛ of an inch; others hang down for several inches. There is no one way that a vulva, let alone the labia minora, is supposed to look. The shapes of the labia minora also vary, and it's this very part that frames the vaginal entrance and may lend the vulva the appearance of a seashell, heart, or flower.

The labia minora are filled with blood vessels and therefore deepen in color, swell slightly, and increase bloodflow to the genitals when a woman is sexually aroused. Some women find that they like to gently tug on or stroke their labia majora or minora during self-pleasuring or partner play. Other women even claim that they ask their partners to gently nibble on their labia minora when things get hot.

Between the labia minora is the **vaginal entrance,** the size of which can vary slightly from woman to woman. Note that this

"It Hurts"

Approximately 10 to 15 percent of women experience pain at their vaginal entrance due to a condition called vulvodynia, which means "vulvar pain." That's an enormous number of women! The pain may come and go, or it may be chronic and ongoing. It might burn, itch, sting, or feel like a stabbing pain. Women may feel pain on their vulva while sitting, driving, riding a bicycle, or during self-pleasuring or partner sex. If you feel discomfort or pain on your vulva or inside your vagina, please contact the National Vulvodynia Association (www.nva.org) for more information, and check in with your healthcare provider.

is not the vagina itself—it is just the entrance—and it is also sometimes called the vaginal opening or, including the area around it, the vestibule. Sometimes women with a condition called localized vulvodynia may experience redness, inflammation, or pain around this area. (See "It Hurts" on page 35.)

The clitoris, urethra, and vagina are so interconnected that stimulation or movement of one is likely to affect the other two parts. As such, Dr. O'Connell has recently suggested that the clitoris, urethra, and vagina be considered a "unit" and perhaps be referred to as the **clitoral complex**. However these parts are described in scientific circles, the take-home messages in terms of sex and pleasure are these:

✱ Vaginal stimulation (whether with fingers, toys, or a penis) can indirectly stimulate the clitoris, as may other types of genital touching.

✱ The interconnectedness of the clitoris, vagina, and urethra may contribute to how women experience sex, such as why some women feel as though they need to urinate while they are having sex (even if their bladder is empty).

✱ Because the clitoris is larger than it appears and extends into the body, there are various direct and indirect ways to stimulate one's clitoris, either privately or with a partner. Such techniques are discussed in Chapter 8.

The **perineum** is the area of skin that lies between the bottom of the vulva and the anal opening. Sometimes people refer to it as the "tween," as it is be*tween* these two parts. Women who have given birth vaginally may know that this area is vulnerable to natural tearing during childbirth and may sometimes be surgically cut during labor in a procedure known as an episiotomy. This procedure has become less widely practiced than it once was, as new research suggests that episiotomies tend to not heal as well as natural tearing. Sometimes, however, an episiotomy may be medically necessary; talk to your healthcare provider if you are pregnant and have questions about the possibility of an episiotomy during your delivery.

Now that you know the parts, let's take a look at some drawings of vulvas so you can get a sense of how widely they can vary in appearance (see below). If you catch yourself feeling uncomfortable, that's okay. Take note of that feeling. If a negative reaction keeps you from experiencing interest or feeling comfortable while learning about your body, it might be something to think about later on. Explore where the negative feelings are coming from. If you find that you're feeling curious, that's okay, too. Again, some women have never seen their own vulva, let alone a stranger's. Curiosity is natural and, I think, should be encouraged. After all, this is the body in which you'll live your whole life. Why not get to know it?

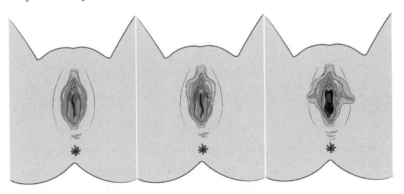

Women's vulvar parts come in a variety of shapes and sizes— there is no "standard."

Note the differences in the shapes and sizes of the labia and clitoral hoods. Though you can't see the differences in color here, parts of the vulva can be varying shades of pink, brown, red, white, gray, black, or peach. Now, if you're feeling less alone or if you're thinking that it's kind of cool that nature gave us these amazing body parts that are basically there to help us feel good, that reassurance or interest is a pleasure, too. Embrace it.

THE HAIR DOWN THERE

Though we won't spend too much time on the topic of pubic hair, I think it's worth at least a few words, given changing trends affecting this area of our bodies. Over the past few years it seems like countless magazines featured articles about Brazilian bikini waxes and detailing how to go "bare." *Sex and the City* featured Brazilian waxing in an episode, and the whole world got a peek at the wax jobs of Britney Spears, Paris Hilton, and Lindsay Lohan on various Hollywood gossip Web sites.

The fact is that not as many women wax off all of their hair as you might expect—and many women and men prefer for their partner to have at least *some* hair down there (albeit often trimmed or groomed). Some women find it extremely pleasurable to keep some amount of pubic hair both for looks and for feel. During self-pleasuring, women may find that they like to run their fingertips through their pubic hair or even to tug slightly on it. Then again, other women prefer the smooth, hairless feel of a bare vulva. There is no right or wrong choice. However, I want to encourage you to consider the following when you're wondering what to do with the hair down there.

✳ How do *you*—not only your partner, but you!—like for your vulva to look? What makes you feel sexy and desirable?

✳ How do you like for your vulva to feel?

✳ How does having (or not having) pubic hair affect how you feel during sex in terms of comfort or pleasure?

✳ What feels like the safest method of pubic hair styling for you? If you have sensitive skin or are prone to irritation or allergy, check in with your healthcare provider for advice on hair removal.

✳ What fits within your budget? After all, feeling stretched for cash or anxious about money can have a dampening effect on anyone's sex drive—and hair removal can be expensive.

Of course, no method of hair removal is perfect. Some women have an unfortunate knack for nicking themselves with a razor, and trust me, cuts on one's vulva never feel good. Other women are allergic to wax and may break out or develop ongoing irritation from being waxed. Others are prone to skin discoloration from laser hair reduction. Whether you choose to go *au naturel* or to trim, groom, or remove your pubic hair, focus on what works for you—not what your sister, best friend, or a celebrity does.

If you are considering pubic hair removal, ask a healthcare provider, such as a dermatologist, for information or advice. Some methods are better suited to women who have certain skin types or who are from certain racial or ethnic backgrounds, given the different ways that our hair follicles develop. You can read a little bit about this in *The V Book: A Doctor's Guide to Complete Vulvovaginal Health* by Elizabeth G. Stewart, MD, and Paula Spencer.

THE VAGINA

The vagina is not, as you now know, the same as the vulva. The word "vagina" refers to a woman's birth canal—the inside part through which babies pass, menstrual blood flows, tampons may be inserted, or sexual penetration with a penis, fingers, or a sex toy may be enjoyed. The vagina can be a mighty busy place—fortunately, all of this stuff does not happen at once. The vagina is less of a multitasker and more like a jack-of-all-trades.

The vagina is usually described as a fibromuscular tube, which isn't quite accurate. The vagina is surrounded by muscles, but it isn't quite "tubelike." Researchers have identified five different vaginal shapes among women, some of which are more prevalent among women from certain racial or ethnic backgrounds. (If you can believe it, they identified these shapes by making internal casts of women's vaginas!) These shapes have been given the following names: parallel, conical, pumpkin seed, heart, and slug (see opposite page). More research needs to be conducted in this area, but some researchers believe that vaginal shape may account for a woman's preference for specific kinds of menstrual products, or methods of birth control, or their experience of pain during intercourse.

Smell and Taste

Many women worry about their vaginal smell and taste. In most cases, women's vaginas smell just fine—possibly a little sweet or yeasty, but that's normal. If your vaginal discharge smells foul or fishy, check in with your healthcare provider, as that may indicate a bacterial imbalance or a vaginal infection. My research suggests[2] that worrying about one's vaginal smell or taste may interfere with a woman's ability to orgasm, so as long as your vagina is healthy, try to relax and learn to enjoy your body's natural scents.

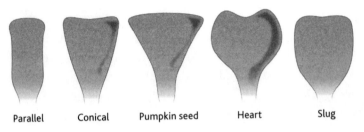

| Parallel | Conical | Pumpkin seed | Heart | Slug |

Women's vagina shapes

If you have ever inserted a finger into your vagina, you know that the mucosal tissue that lines the vagina feels soft and wet. The vagina is basically its own little world—it likes to maintain a specific pH level (a measure of how acidic or alkaline something is), and if that pH is thrown off, it is often a sign of an imbalance or infection. (A quick test by your healthcare provider can reveal your vaginal pH.) Because the vaginal environment is sensitive, the vagina is generally not fond of feminine hygiene products (such as douches, sprays, or powders) or scented soaps or body washes, all of which can throw off the vaginal pH or cause irritation or itching. You do not need to clean the vagina. It actually cleans itself. Just like our eyes clean themselves with teardrops and the discharge we wipe out of the corners of our eyes each morning, the vagina uses vaginal discharge to keep itself clean. Women vary in terms of their natural vaginal discharge—some women feel fairly wet and others feel fairly dry. This can change throughout the menstrual cycle, in response to certain medications, and over the course of a woman's life. If you have questions about your vaginal discharge, ask your healthcare provider so that your worries won't get in the way of your ability to enjoy your body and experience pleasure.

Let's look at some of the unique characteristics of the vagina and how they contribute to the experience of sexual

•

pleasure. First, let's talk size. I am so tired of people talking about "loose vaginas." Amazingly enough, women's vaginas seem to bounce back in terms of their size and shape even after they have been stretched due to childbirth. In a 1996 study,[3] no significant differences in vaginal size were found between women who had never given birth and those who had delivered one or more babies. That said, some women may notice changes in wetness, elasticity, or sensation as they age—all of which can be addressed with one's healthcare provider or sex therapist.

But when it comes to size, whether it is penis or vaginal size, I try to encourage women and men to think more in terms of genital fit than vaginal or penile size. Sure, there are different vaginal sizes and shapes, but they're not dramatically different. In the aforementioned study, women who were measured for vaginal size ranged in width (probably the closest metric we can use to measure perceived "tightness" or "looseness") from 4.8 cm to 6.3 cm. That's only a difference of one and a half centimeters! Given that we already subject our waists, hips, breasts, and thighs to constant measurement, can we at least leave the vagina alone?

If, during intercourse, you experience a lack of feeling, it may be because you are so amazingly wet and well lubricated—which is a good thing! To feel more sensation, try using a towel to dab off some of the natural lubrication from your vaginal entrance—just the outside part—and from your partner's penis or the sex toy you're using, and then return to sex. You may then feel "tighter" or more sensitive. On the other hand, if you feel too tight during intercourse, which is common if you don't spend much time in foreplay or if you jump into sex after getting out of a warm bath or shower, try using a store-bought lubricant. Lubrication has far more to do with our own and our partner's perceptions of vaginal size than our actual bodies do.

Besides, vaginal size changes. Most vaginas tend to be 3 to 4 inches long when a woman is not aroused. But when she starts feeling aroused or excited, the vagina does the most amazing thing: It "tents." Muscular tension pulls the uterus upward, which makes the vaginal canal expand in both length and width, making more room for fingers, a sex toy, or a partner's penis. Seriously—check out the diagrams on page 44. (And turn to Chapter 4 to learn more about tenting and arousal.)

Given that a man's penis averages 5 to 6 inches long when

Sex Ed

Vaginal tightening creams are commonly sold in many adult bookstores and on adult Web sites. However, many formulas tend to work by causing inflammation (and swelling) of the vaginal tissue—the inflammation is what causes the vagina to feel tighter. Ouch! Who wants to irritate and inflame their vagina? Not me. If you want a safer way to feel more sensation during intercourse, try using the towel trick (described on the opposite page) or time your sex accordingly. For example, if you rely on intense stimulation for orgasm, slip into your most orgasm-prone positions either in the early stages of intercourse (before you've had a chance to lubricate that much) or late in the game (if you're having marathon sex sessions, as lubrication may subside with time). Doing regular Kegel exercises (see page 186 for a how-to) can also help you learn to contract the muscles around your vagina in ways that heighten sensation and increase your pleasure. That said, some women find that they experience unusually high amounts of vaginal lubrication and that the best strategy for them is to briefly insert a tampon (for 10 to 30 seconds), then remove it before resuming sex. By absorbing lubrication, you may find a more sensitive and pleasurable balance of wetness.

erect, it's a good thing that the vagina grows a few inches longer to make room for an average-size penis. It is also a good thing that penis enlargement pills and herbs don't really work. There is only so much a woman can fit into her vagina, and as wondrous as vaginas are, most are simply not built to comfortably fit 9, 10, or more inches of an erect penis inside.

If you find that sex feels uncomfortable, try spending more time in foreplay to kick your vaginal tenting (and natural vaginal lubrication) into gear, thus making more room in your vagina. You can also add a store-bought lubricant to your own or your partner's genitals for more comfortable, pleasurable sex.

Another interesting tidbit about the vagina is that it is not nearly as nerve-dense as the glans clitoris. This surprises many

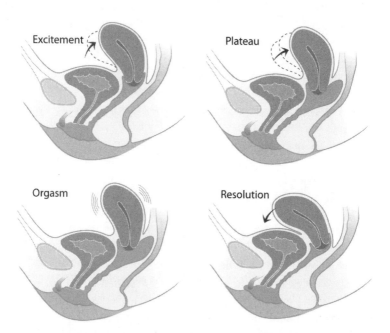

Vaginal changes during sexual stimulation

people who wonder, then, why it feels good to have sex or how women can orgasm through vaginal intercourse if the glans clitoris is not inside the vagina. The answer is that just because the vagina is not as densely packed with nerve endings as the clitoris is does not mean that the vagina isn't sensitive to touch or deep pressure. In the groundbreaking 1953 publication *Sexual Behavior in the Human Female*, pioneering sexuality researcher Dr. Alfred Kinsey and his team noted that although few women stimulated their vagina during masturbation (most focused on the clitoris, as women still do today), many still enjoyed vaginal stimulation, particularly with a partner, with some noting that deep vaginal pressure felt most pleasurable. Keep in mind, of course, that we now know that vaginal intercourse may indirectly stimulate those inside parts of the clitoris (the crura), which are highly sensitive and that, as the crura are composed of erectile tissue, they swell during sexual arousal (making them similar to the inside parts of a man's penis, which also swell during arousal). As such, the clitoris is intrinsically linked with most women's experiences of sexual pleasure.

Sex Ed

Did you know that the vagina actually sits at an angle of about 130° in an unaroused state?

When the vagina tents during sexual arousal, the uterus tips upward, which helps to elongate the vagina and minimize the angle. As a woman ages and her muscle tone weakens, the angle of the vagina tends to flatten. This change in angle, in addition to declining levels of vaginal lubrication, partly explains why sex feels different with age—not necessarily worse, but certainly different.

THE G-SPOT

The G-spot is an area of the vagina named, in 1987, after Dr. Ernst Grafenberg. In 1950, Dr. Grafenberg had described an area along the front wall of the vagina (1 or 2 inches inside) that, when stimulated, felt pleasurable to some but not all women (see below).

Like any other part of a woman's body (including the glans clitoris), the G-spot is not a magic button. Sometimes the G-spot is unfairly touted as something that, if it could only be found by women and their partners, would make everything great. Sex, like life, is more complex than that. (However, I will certainly share more about the G-spot with you—including techniques for private exploration and partner play—in Chapter 8.)

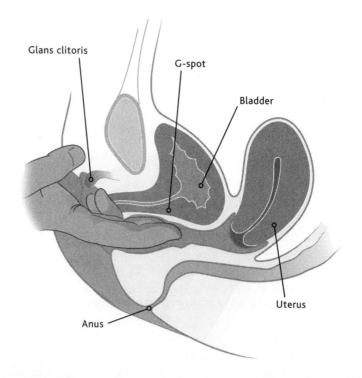

Glans clitoris

G-spot

Bladder

Uterus

Anus

Do some women experience arousing sensations when their G-spot is stimulated? Yes, but not everyone does, and that's okay. Not all women enjoy direct stimulation of the clitoris or light tugging of one's pubic hairs or stroking of the labia, either. The magic of our sexual experiences lies in the fact that we are all so similar and yet so different.

So why do some women like how it feels for their G-spot to be touched or stimulated? To be honest, scientists are not entirely certain. One common theory, however, is that G-spot stimulation actually stimulates the erectile tissue surrounding the urethra (the tube that carries urine from the bladder and out of the body) on the other side of the vaginal wall or the urethral bulbs on either side of the urethra. Another thought is that G-spot stimulation may actually be stimulating the crura (again, as part of the "clitoral complex," which means that stimulation of one part—such as the front wall of the vagina— stimulates another part). In any case, one thing is clear:

Good-Bye, UTI

Have you ever wondered whether drinking cranberry juice can really help defeat a urinary tract infection (UTI)? What the research shows is that drinking cranberry juice can help to *prevent* UTIs—however, the jury is still out on whether it can help to *treat* a UTI. Be careful if you go the cranberry juice route, though, as you'd have to drink a large amount of cranberry juice (and drink it every day) for maximum effectiveness, which would translate into loads of calories—and thus extra pounds. Instead, try drinking unsweetened cranberry juice concentrate mixed with water, or ask your healthcare provider about taking cranberry juice concentrate tablets, which have also been shown to be effective at preventing UTIs for some women.[4]

Because the G-spot area is not rich with nerve endings, it is therefore not sensitive to light touch (as the glans clitoris is). Whatever is being stimulated—whether it's the erectile tissue around the urethra, the urethral bulbs, or the crura—responds best to gentle yet firm pressure, which likely has to be just firm enough to rub things the right way on the other side of the front vaginal wall.

FACT: *It's possible to be allergic to semen.*

Strange but true—though first documented in 1958, there are now at least 80 scientifically documented cases of human seminal plasma allergy (HSPA). Symptoms may range from slight itching, redness, or irritation on the vulva or in the vagina (from exposure to semen during intercourse) to, more severely, shortness of breath, dizziness, or nausea. If you suspect that you're allergic to semen, please discuss your symptoms with your healthcare provider. While mild cases of HSPA may inhibit pleasure, more severe cases can put your health at risk.

MYTH: *Vaginas are dirty.*

Au contraire! Vaginas are self-cleaning and, thanks to a relatively steady stream of natural vaginal and cervical discharge, our vaginas are kept quite clean, thank you very much. Unless your healthcare provider advises you otherwise, there is no need to douche or to use a feminine hygiene spray, wipe, powder, or deodorant—all of which can cause vaginal or vulvar itching, burning, or irritation. Plus, as Eve Ensler wrote in her award-winning play *The Vagina Monologues*, "My vagina doesn't need to be cleaned up. It smells good already."

HOMEWORK
Vulvar Self-Examination:
The Basics

Now that we've checked out diagrams and drawings of other women's vulvas, I'm going to ask you to look at your own vulva. In the next day or two, I'd like for you to do the following homework exercise as you learn to perform a vulvar self-examination. The purpose of this is to learn to identify the parts of your vulva, to get comfortable looking at and touching your parts, and to become familiar with what is normal for you. Again, since there is no one "standard" vulva, the important issue in terms of your health is finding out what is typical for *you*.

1. First, find some private time when you feel relaxed, fully at ease, and unlikely to be interrupted. Whether that means that you first go for a run, soak in a warm bath, or drop your iPod in the docking station and listen to your favorite music is up to you.

2. Take out a hand mirror or large compact mirror and get comfortable in a well-lit area of your home. This may be sitting on your bed or on the floor, or standing with one leg propped up on a chair or the toilet seat.

3. Open your legs enough to be able to see your vulva. Identify your mons and labia majora. If you have pubic hair, look through it to your skin and check for any freckles, moles, or bumps. Also notice the color of your skin underneath your hair, which is likely very similar to the shade of the skin that covers most of your body.

4. Now look for your clitoral hood and glans clitoris. Notice how sensitive it likely feels to the touch, particularly if you try to move the hood back away from the glans clitoris. (That hood is there for a reason!) There may be a small amount of smegma—white or grayish "stuff" that is composed of dead skin cells and oil from your skin. Some women occasionally pull their clitoral hood back to brush away the smegma. The glans clitoris may be similar to or different in color than most of your body's skin. It may be pink, gray, black, peach, brown, or similar shades. Don't expect to find anything green or blue or gold, however—it's not that exciting. *(continued)*

HOMEWORK—CONTINUED

5. Next, identify your labia minora and check out their size, shape, and most likely their lack of symmetry. (Most of us do not have perfectly symmetrical labia.) What do yours look like? Do they resemble a seashell, flower, heart, or angel wings? Are they big, medium, or petite? What color are they? Is the color uniform all over, or does the shading vary? What is the texture like? Again, the skin tone of your labia minora is likely different than that of your other body parts.

6. Check out your vaginal entrance, which may be slightly more pink or red for some women. Does it feel comfortable or uncomfortable to touch around the entrance?

Now that you've identified the parts of the vulva, make a mental note of what your vulva looks like in terms of the color, size, and shape of each part. Let your healthcare provider know if you would like more information, and feel free to ask questions about any changes you notice in terms of color, texture, and feeling (such as developing spots or patches of white skin, or areas that feel uncomfortable or painful to touch). You should perform a vulvar self-examination about once per month so that you're aware of any changes and can consult with a healthcare provider as needed. Sometimes you may find lumps, bumps, or freckles on your vulva—these do not necessarily signal anything bad. In fact, they're fairly common. But it is always a good idea to let your healthcare provider know what you find during your self-examinations.

Now that you know the parts of the vulva, consider touching each of them in soft versus more firm ways, or in quick versus slow rhythms with your fingertips. Which parts feel more or less sensitive? Which parts feel pleasurable when touched? What feels good, intriguing, or uncomfortable?

Becoming familiar with your vulva is an important part of exploring your body in ways that bring you and your partner pleasure. It also enhances your ability to accurately communicate symptoms to your healthcare provider. Now if you have an itch that doesn't go away, you can say, "I have an itch on my right labium," rather than, "It itches down there."

Cultivating Desire

Learning to Want Sex Again

When we are in danger of losing something to which we've become accustomed, we may suddenly realize its value and want it even more. Such is the case with love and lust. These feelings offer us an enormous amount of pleasure, but it's easy to lose sight of their importance in our lives—until they are gone. This chapter is about gently coaxing desire from its hiding place. While we all have the capacity to experience desire, at times we become sorely disconnected from it and may begin to feel more apathetic than passionate. Evelyn Resh, a colleague whose work I admire, studies the connection between sexuality and sensuality. As director of Sexual Health Services for Canyon Ranch, in the Berkshires, she cautions against a disconnection of these two principles, stating that, "the more detached we become from life's

•

pleasures . . . the more fatigue and sensual atrophy we will experience. And with that, our libidinal energy will plummet, leaving us marooned in the land of 'No': no time, no energy, no opportunity, no sex." And I would add: no desire. Ready to change that?

POP QUIZ

1. Which of the following commonly contribute to low or inhibited desire?

    a. Depression
    b. Relationship problems
    c. Poor body image
    d. Unpleasurable sexual experiences
    e. All of the above

2. Approximately what percentage of couples have experienced sexual problems?

    a. 10 to 20%
    b. 32 to 40%
    c. 57 to 70%
    d. 78 to 95%

3. Which of the following is least likely to decline substantially with age?

    a. Vaginal lubrication
    b. Sexual satisfaction
    c. Sexual desire
    d. None of the above; they all decline substantially with age

4. True or False: Low testosterone is responsible for most cases of low desire among women.

5. Which of the following is most likely to make sex more pleasurable for a person or couple?

    a. Strong erections

    b. Vaginal orgasms

    c. Physical and psychological relaxation

    d. Increased vaginal lubrication

    e. None of the above

Answers: 1) e; 2) d; 3) b; 4) False; 5) c

Most people, at some point in their lives, will experience a decrease in—or even a total loss of—sexual desire or interest. Perhaps you used to readily hop into bed with your partner or vibrator in the middle of the day, and you no longer do. Or maybe you're easily excited about sex these days, but you recall a stretch of time when you would have rather read a book, cooked a good meal, taken a walk, or gone directly and soundly to sleep. It is common to experience ups and downs in your level of desire over time—and it makes sense, too. After all, if everyone stayed in bed and had sex multiple times a day, what would we ever accomplish as a society? Who would raise our children, care for aging parents, go to work, or clean the house?

Not only is it common and healthy to experience occasional ups and downs in your level of desire, but it can feel reinvigorating when you find—after either a short or prolonged dry spell—that your capacity for pleasurable, satisfying, inspiring sex didn't completely go away, though it may temporarily have gone into hiding. In this chapter, I want you to learn how to:

✳ Become more gentle, accepting, patient—and even curious—about your own and your partner's experiences of desire

* Be able to identify at least one or two factors that support your ability to both feel and express your desires

* Learn or rediscover at least one form of touch that feels good on your body (or that you'd like to use on another person's body)

* Try talking to your partner (if you have one) about each other's desires and how they work in your relationship

* Feel confident that you can make changes to enhance your desire if yours feels low in a way that bothers you

THE FIRST BLUSH OF DESIRE

Think of a time when you absolutely reveled in your sexual desire. I don't care whether it was for a moment or an hour, or whether you acted on it or not; I simply would like for you to think about a moment—recently or in the past—when you let yourself bask in the depths and the pleasures of your desire. Perhaps you remember returning to school one fall to find that a fellow student who never stood out had blossomed over the summer into someone whom you couldn't take your eyes off of. Or maybe you remember hanging out with someone or going on dates, hoping each time that "good-bye" would lead to a kiss, a grope, or hours in bed. Maybe you remember how long you stood there, waiting to be kissed or to find the right moment to kiss someone. You may even recall the electricity you felt in your body when your crush touched your back, held your hand, or looked at you a certain way.

For those who have been in one or more long-term relationships, you might remember being at a party, bar, or

Cuing Desire

These simple activities are designed to jump-start your desire and are based on the idea that sexual stimuli can cause your body to become physically aroused, which can, in turn, encourage desire. Try any of the following to see if they enhance your experience or expression of desire. (See Resources on page 234 for book and film suggestions.)

* Read sexy stories, such as romance novels or erotica.

* Read suggestive or romantic poetry to your partner while lying in bed.

* Watch sexually explicit films together or privately.

* Take turns drawing pictures of things you would like to do with each other.

* Allow your mind to indulge in sexual fantasies during the day, or as you drift off to sleep.

* Remember why you fell in love with your partner, what initially attracted you to each other, and situations in which you have felt highly aroused by him or her.

* Stimulate your genitals with your hand or vibrator (on a low intensity).

* Display affection for your partner with kisses, hugs, touches, and massage.

* Write out a fantasy that feels exciting to you—it doesn't have to be anything you would ever do in real life.

* Exercise in a way that puts you in touch with your body or helps you feel sexy, such as salsa dancing, running, pole dancing, belly dancing, or yoga.

* Schedule a sexual or sensual activity (such as a massage or bathing together) with your partner and build up excitement and desire throughout the day by calling each other or by sending affectionate Facebook messages or racy text messages.

at home with your family, and suddenly you looked across the room and saw your partner shine in a way you hadn't noticed in quite some time. Maybe he was smiling and talking with his friends, reading a story to your children, or ordering a meal from the waiter in a foreign language. Maybe he was simply stepping out of the shower and your heart went, "Wow."

In the space below, I want you to jot down three times that you have experienced desire in a way that felt good to you. A quick description will do, such as "First day of school in 11th grade/Craig Smith." I just want you to have something to come back to if you forget, sometime in the future, what desire can feel like. You can always return to this page, read your notes, and think carefully about the circumstances that prompted you to feel such intense desire. If you've never or rarely experienced desire in a pleasurable way, and you want to, rest assured that you can make positive changes. Ready?

THREE DESIRE-RICH MOMENTS

1.

_____

_____

_____

2.

_____

_____

_____

3.

_____

_____

_____

Desire's Ups and Downs

We hear so much about low desire that we may lose sight of how natural it is for desire to ebb and flow. Sometimes desire may feel strong and effortless (and often does when one is young); at other times, mustering any desire at all may feel enormously difficult. Most of the time, however, desire exists somewhere in the middle rather than at either extreme.

In spite of what we hear about low desire, it isn't always a bad thing. Many sexual health professionals suspect that it can even be a reflection of the wise workings of the mind-body connection. For example, if you have recently had a baby, then your needs are well served by caring for your baby or getting sleep and a shower. If you're going through menopause, then both your body and mind are adjusting to a variety of new feelings and sensations, as well as mood and temperature changes, not to mention sexual and vaginal changes.

It can take time to adjust to life changes or interruptions, and sometimes, by experiencing changes in desire, your body may be taking care of you intuitively. With time, patience, and some care and attention, your desire may return on its own. Then again, sometimes it doesn't. Sometimes it feels like there is nothing we can do to make ourselves feel interested in sex. Other times we do feel sexually interested, but not in our partners. Often, however, desire remains alive underneath the surface (yes, even when you think it's gone for good)—and yet we may feel unsure, timid, hesitant, or embarrassed about *expressing* our desire. This is what we sometimes call "inhibited desire."

Desire Disruptors

Many factors can disrupt a person's experience or expression of desire. Here are a few common issues that may contribute to decreased desire.

✳ **Depression.** Even mild depression has been associated with low desire—as have some of the medications that are used to treat it. Fortunately, counseling is effective for many cases of depression, as are lifestyle changes such as diet, rest, and exercise. A wide range of medications—including some with little, if any, risk of sexual side effects—are also available by prescription. Talk to your healthcare provider or a therapist if you feel unusually anxious, sad, or angry.

✳ **Unpleasurable sexual experiences.** If your experience of sex has not felt good either in general or with a particular person, it is understandable (and expected) that you would not be very interested in having more sex. It is normal for people to want to avoid things that have been unpleasant. Luckily, even if your past experiences haven't been enjoyable, there are ways to create pleasurable sex with that same partner.

✳ **Health conditions, medications, hormonal issues, and surgical treatments.** Various health conditions including hypertension, thyroid problems, diabetes, and cancer have been linked to low levels of desire, as have various medications (including some oral contraceptives and sedatives) and surgical treatments (such as hysterectomy). In addition, some medications (such as antidepressants) may have sexual side effects that can result in vaginal dryness, decreased desire, or difficulty experiencing orgasm. Although hormonal changes themselves are rarely responsible for low sexual desire, it is possible. Talk to your doctor if you're concerned that hormonal issues may be affecting your desire.

✳ **Past assault, rape, molestation, or abuse.** Unfortunately, many women (and men) have been sexually, physically, or emotionally assaulted or abused as adults, or were molested as children. Sexual touching as an adult can trigger painful memories related to the earlier trauma. Moving past these experiences can take time and is often helped by the support and guidance of a professional (see Resources on page 234).

✳ **Negative messages about one's sexuality or body.** Some women were told, as girls, that touching their bodies was "dirty" or "bad." Others, as teenagers or adults, were called "sluts" or "tramps" by people whom they cared about and whose opinions mattered to them. As an adult, you may still initially experience feelings of guilt, shame, or embarrassment in relation to your sexual feelings or behavior. Turning negative self-talk around (see Chapter 1) can be helpful, as can challenging your thinking on these types of beliefs. It's often true that old beliefs have to fall away to make room for new ones.

✳ **Concerns about pregnancy or infection.** If a woman is concerned about becoming pregnant or getting a sexually transmissible disease (STD), she is unlikely to desire sex. That may seem obvious, but it is often overlooked when considering the roots of inhibited desire. Talk to your healthcare provider to learn about reliable methods of contraception that may be available to you (see Resources on page 234).

Other common contributors to low or inhibited desire may include poor body image, concerns about aging, self-consciousness, anxiety about being a skilled lover, concerns about being "used," feeling unable to "let go" in front of one's partner, or not feeling attracted to one's partner. Later in this chapter you will find additional ideas to consider (and activities to try) that may help you to feel better able and equipped to express desire in ways that feel good.

Desire Discrepancy

First, however, we should acknowledge one of the most common difficulties related to desire, and that is when both partners have some level of desire and they want to have sex with each other, yet not with the same level of frequency or in the same way. This "desire discrepancy," as it is often called, can lead to one or both people questioning their sexual, if not overall, compatibility as a couple. Maybe one person wants sex to last for 30 minutes and the other prefers quicker sex. Or else it's about adventure or variety—one partner wants to try toys, new positions, or threesomes, and the other is happy with their sex life as is. Often the issue is centered around the frequency of

Sex Ed

If it has been awhile since you have had or initiated sex with your partner, or if you have experienced a lot of hurt or pain in your relationship, it can take some time to experience desire again and to reconnect sexually. Allow yourself to take baby steps. Rather than focusing on initiating sex, try to initiate hand-holding, eye contact, kisses, back rubs, or cuddles on the couch. If you're concerned that your partner may jump the gun and pressure you for sex, let him or her know what you're up to—and that you're trying—but that you'd like some space to take things slowly.

sex: One person wants to have sex three times a week, and the other would be happy having sex once or twice a month. These differences are not, as is often assumed, necessarily related to gender—sometimes men want more frequent sex, and at other times, women do. And the e-mails and letters I get from people who are seeking help are not always from the partner who is trying to figure out how to get more sex. Sometimes I hear from men or women who are looking for ways to "tame" their desire, so as not to feel like they are bothering or pressuring their partner for more sex than they want to have.

In fact, it is quite common for two people who love each other to have different levels of desire. After all, what are the chances that we'll meet someone who has all of the characteristics we want in a relationship partner (such as they're smart, kind, funny, honest, trusting, reliable, and easygoing), who we are in love with, attracted to, share similar values and goals with, and who just happens to have *exactly* the same sex drive we do? Even if you are lucky enough to find such a perfect mate, life throws us all curveballs—a new job that is stressful, babies that require night feedings, or an illness that fatigues us— which can alter how we think and feel about sex.

Given the enormous potential for differences in desire between two people, it is no surprise that although about half of women and men are said to be experiencing significant sexual problems at any given time, the vast majority of couples (some suggest 78 to 95 percent) experience occasional sexual problems that may not be severe enough to be considered "dysfunctional" but that can cause the sorts of disagreements and issues that many can identify with: arguments about masturbation, pornography, attraction, emotional needs, and how long sex should ideally last. Considering this enormous range of sexual problems and disagreements, it is fair to ask whether this so-called "desire discrepancy" is perhaps better described as an opportunity for couples to figure out how to negotiate a sex life with each other in a way that feels good to both people involved.

Cultivating Desire

While many women experience desire effortlessly (spontaneous desire) when they are young or in new or very passionate, high-chemistry relationships, the experience of desire may be different for some women as they age, stay in a long-term relationship, or deal with stressors or health issues. At times, women (and, I would argue, men, too) feel as though they need to make a special effort to cultivate desire, or that they need certain "preconditions" to be met before they feel, or express, their desire—such as feeling relaxed and emotionally connected with their partner.

In long-term relationships this may be particularly true, as it is rarely the case that women don't want to have sex with their partner any longer, but rather the issue is that that the bar gets raised. Early on, having a fun night out at dinner, sharing laughs, realizing you have the same taste in music, and mutual attraction may be enough to turn you on. As your relationship progresses, however, you may need more from your partner in order to want sex. Now that you're familiar with each other, thinking about shared interests or fun experiences probably isn't enough to sexually excite you. Instead, you may need to feel like your partner desires you—not just because you are "available" (the relationship version of "easy"), but because there is something unique, special, and beautiful about you. Time and again, research suggests that in order for women to experience

desire, they first need to feel that they are desired both physically and emotionally—perhaps not all of the time, but certainly
a good amount of the time—and that they are respected and
treated like equals in their relationship.

Expressing Desire

But sometimes desire isn't enough. Many people experience
feelings of desire for their partner but don't act on them. In my
work, I've found it helpful to encourage both women and men to
consider the factors that make it easier to express their desire
to one another. What do you need in order to feel like you could
initiate sex or respond to a partner's advances in receptive,
pleasurable ways? Many women are more comfortable expressing desire when one or more of the following emotional needs
are met.

* They feel safe or cared for by a partner.

* They believe they are attractive, wanted, desired, or sexy.

* They feel respected, admired, or understood by a
  partner.

* They're able to relax and experience sex free from
  disruption.

Do you identify with any of these needs? What other "keys to
desire" are important to you?

Because desire is largely a psychological experience, many
women find that it is critical for them to first face issues of
their own or their partner's expectations, ideas about sex,
communication styles, and varying abilities to relax. Attend-
ing to the mind-body connection in this way can help to make
sex feel more *pleasurable*. And if you can figure out how to make

sex feel good more often, then you are probably going to want it more often!

Consider the ideas below, and think about which ones might be helpful to you.

- ✻ **Set realistic expectations.** Considering that even sexually satisfied couples only have sex that they would call "very good" about one out of every four or five times (20 to 25 percent of the time), is it fair to expect that every sex act should be "mind-blowing"? Of course not! Have positive—but realistic—expectations about what sex can feel like so that you are likely to enjoy it, rather than feel disappointed. That way, you're sure to want more of it another time.

- ✻ **Be fair about your bodies.** Similarly, work on developing fair and realistic expectations about your body and your partner's body. A 50-year-old man is unlikely to have an erection that is as rigid, or as easy to come by, as a man half his age would; likewise, a woman is unlikely to have breasts that are as perky at age 40 as they were at age 20, particularly if she has breastfed. Expectations about bodies and sexual function that are appropriate to one's age and life experiences are key to feeling good about sex and enhancing one's desire, particularly given that some women and men find that their desire is inhibited by concerns about their bodies not being "perfect" or like the airbrushed images in advertisements and movies.

- ✻ **Examine your stereotypes.** In order to fit in with society's version of a "good girl," many women feel pressured to avoid sex, to shy away from initiating it even when they want to, to not masturbate (or at least to never admit to it), and to suppress expressions of their sexual feelings. As a reflection of these stereotypes, in a 2006 study conducted by researchers from the California Institute of Technology, young college women were found to be more likely to talk about sex in terms of fear or anxiety (such as about infection or pregnancy risk) than about pleasure. It takes time—sometimes years—for some women to feel sexually comfortable in their own skin. Giving yourself permission to enjoy your sexuality, and to create your own definitions of what it means to be a sexually confident and experienced woman, may help to enhance your desire and your experience of sex.

✳ **Talk to each other.** Just as women and men may have unfair stereotypes about their own gender, many have unfair stereotypes about the opposite sex, too. As an example, in a 2004 study of 152 heterosexual couples, researchers from the University of New Brunswick found that women often underestimated how long their partners wanted to spend in foreplay and intercourse. This is really too bad, because when individuals operate on assumptions without checking in with their partner, they run the risk of doing something that neither one of them enjoys. They may also be missing out on a sexual activity (or a night off from having sex) that both would welcome.

✳ **Relax.** You'll find me saying this multiple times throughout this book, and for good reason: It. Is. Critical. Mental and physical relaxation cultivate a supportive environment in which sexual intimacy can flourish.

Relaxation makes it easier for men to have erections, for women to lubricate (and orgasm), and for members of both genders to feel open to sexual pleasure, intimacy, and desire. In the 1970s, sex research pioneers Masters and Johnson found that relaxation could work magic on sexual function and desire (one of the many reasons why desire may peak while you're on vacation!). They created a set of exercises called "sensate focus" that encourages relaxation and touching among couples (see page 70). Try to take time in your lovemaking and to approach it with a calm, centered, present mind.

✳ **Play!** Couples who play together, stay together—or at least they often have satisfying sex. Couples dealing with sexual problems tend to exhibit less playfulness. You can change that! If it's been a while since you've had sex, try playing together first in nonsexual ways: Bring out a board game, toss a Frisbee together in the backyard, or play hopscotch as a family. As intimacy grows, turn up the heat on your play: Chase each other around the house, expose your breasts or genitals to your partner during an unexpected moment at home, tickle each other silly and include a few erotic touches, snuggle together on the couch while watching a comedy, wear lingerie, beg dramatically for sex, or sneak off to a beautiful bed-and-breakfast and lock yourselves in your room for an indulgent amount of time. Whether your play is seductive, silly, competitive, or makes your stomach hurt from laughter depends on your personalities and willingness to let go. Just get out there and have fun with each other!

✻ **Be creative.** When a couple is dealing with desire discrepancy, the partner who wants more sex may feel rejected, unattractive, or unwanted. The partner who wants less sex often feels guilty or inadequate for being the holdout. Neither place feels good. Think outside the box: The partner who wants less sex can kiss (or watch) while the other person masturbates, suggest another intimacy-building activity (like taking a bath together or curling up on the couch to watch a movie), or clearly communicate what her or his lack of desire means (see Chapter 1). The partner who wants more sex can learn to take rejection as a no to sex rather than a no to the relationship, and he or she can embrace other sexual or intimacy-building activities.

✻ **Embrace multipurpose sex.** Sometimes people develop low desire because they feel like they and their partner want different things from sex and therefore may be incompatible. However, healthy, satisfied couples often desire sex for different reasons and at different times. Sex may be desired in order to become pregnant, to feel pleasure, to relieve stress, to feel connected, to feel confident about one's relationship, or to have an orgasm. All are real-life reasons and it may be that, at times, you and your partner are having sex with different motivations; that doesn't mean it cannot be physically or emotionally satisfying more of the time.

✻ **Recognize your limits.** Just as it is important to have realistic expectations, it is also critical to recognize how your limits may change with different life stages. As a college student, you may have had fewer responsibilities and all the time in the world to have arousing foreplay and satisfying sex; as a single parent or full-time employee, it may be all you can do to have quickies before sleep during the week and more savory, seductive sex on the weekends. (That is, if your kids are at a sleepover or you're not traveling out of town for work.) Recognizing your own or your partner's limits can free you both from blame and help you think about creative ways to seek pleasure and intimacy in spite of life circumstances.

✳ **Indulge in life's sensual pleasures.** Connecting with your sensuality can help to connect you with your sexuality, including desire. Try any of the following: Walk barefoot in the yard, paying attention to the blades of grass under your feet; arrange fresh flowers, noticing their vibrant color or scent; savor a piece of fruit or glass of wine, paying attention to the flavors in your mouth; kiss someone you adore, such as a partner, friend, family member, or pet, being mindful of their importance in your life.

✳ **Talk some more.** Communicate your needs for feeling comfortable when approaching sex—this may mean telling your partner that you need the space to initiate without feeling pressured or that, for you, foreplay is spending time together talking in the evening, not just climbing into bed and going for it.

✳ **Seek help.** Sometimes sexual or relationship problems have gone on for so long or feel so huge or painful that people don't know where to begin. Rather than wait and hope that it all works out in the end, seek help sooner rather than later. See Resources on page 234 to locate a sex, couples, or marital therapist.

These tips are designed as a smorgasbord—try what feels right to you, come back later for other options, and ignore what doesn't fit with your life. Many desire issues can be helped by feeling more relaxed about sex, being more open to possibilities, addressing relationship issues, and finding a middle ground in desire discrepancies. That said, keep in mind that no one can possibly find the right solution to every problem at once; these suggestions will still be here when you need ideas in the future.

WANTING WHAT YOU HAVE

Many of the tips on the opposite page are connected to the concept of acceptance—which, on a broader level, is a basic tenet of some Eastern philosophies. Buddhist teachers have long instructed their students that contentment comes from wanting what one already has, and dissatisfaction and suffering arise from wanting what one cannot have. This principle holds true for your sex life, too: Happiness and satisfaction result from wanting what one already has.

Most of us have, at some point, bought into an artificial idea of what a great sex life is supposed to look like—a vision that we are unlikely to ever achieve. (And if you do, you might find that it's not all that it's cracked up to be.) The qualifications for this perfect sex life are typically as follows:

✳ Orgasms that are easy to come by (but not too quick!)

✳ For women, orgasms during vaginal intercourse

✳ For men, the ability to last as long as they want (to be able to delay ejaculation) and hard erections that they can get whenever they want

(continued on page 72)

FACT: *Banning sex can be good for you.*

Masters and Johnson developed "sensate focus" exercises that are still commonly used in modern-day sex therapy. In addition, many couples use aspects of these exercises as an informal means of enhancing their desire and their experience of sex. Before couples begin, they generally agree to ban intercourse—or any attempts to stimulate each other's genitals—until they reach the appropriate stages (which may take weeks). When used informally, couples may simply agree to ban sex for a week, a few days, or at least for the 30 minutes or hour that they choose to spend trying these pleasure-focused exercises.

Step 1 involves each partner taking a turn touching the other person's body in ways that feel pleasurable to the one doing the touching. This type of touch is about learning how it feels good to touch and explore another's body—it is not about genital stimulation. In fact, the breasts and genitals should be avoided. The person being touched is encouraged to give feedback about any types of touch that feel bothersome, annoying, or conversely, quite good! A benefit of these exercises is that couples also learn how to express what they like about sensual touching.

Step 2 also involves taking turns touching each other's bodies (again, breasts and genitals excluded); however during this stage, the focus is on the pleasure and enjoyment of the person *receiving* the touch. Again, partners can communicate with each other as to what does or doesn't feel good. Step 3 expands to maintain a focus on pleasure through touch but allows the breasts and genitals to be included. In Step 4, couples continue to use the types of touch that they used in previous steps, but they may also touch each other to the point of orgasm or possibly have intercourse.

Try not to rush through these steps—some couples spend days if not a week or more in each step before moving on to the next. To learn more about these and related exercises, you might enjoy reading *For Each Other: Sharing Sexual Intimacy* by Lonnie Barbach, PhD. If you'd like to try sensate focus exercises with the guidance of a therapist, see Resources on page 234 to find one in your local area.

✗ MYTH: *You should go to bed when you're tired.*

How many times have we heard this piece of advice? And yet, it is only good advice if a person's primary goal is to fall fast asleep. If you are hoping to be sexually intimate with your partner, then head to bed when you still have enough energy to kiss and make out, if not have sex. Then make sure to get a good night's sleep, as feeling tired and fatigued can impact not only your sex life, but also your mood and productivity.

According to a 2007 National Sleep Foundation study, the vast majority of women were regularly running wild during the hour before bed, whether they were cleaning, working, watching television, surfing the Internet, or doing activities with their family. Just imagine if, at least occasionally, you used that wind-down time for sexual intimacy and bonding and for creating a restful space more conducive to sleep. As you consider making your bed a space for both sleep and sex, you might enjoy reading *Two in a Bed*, by Paul Rosenblatt; it explores the intricacies of sharing a bed with another person, including issues of sex, cuddling, stealing sheets and covers, and choosing sides of the bed.

＊ For both, sex that lasts at least 15 minutes, but more often in the 30-minutes to 1-hour range

＊ For men, a large penis

＊ For women, a tight—but not too tight—vagina

＊ For women, adequate wetness (again, not too dry but not too wet)

＊ Frequent sex

＊ Perpetual "readiness" for sex

＊ The ability, for men, to "give" their partner an orgasm

What else would you add to this list of seemingly "idealized" sex traits?

Looking at the above list, it seems that "ideal sex" prizes control and mastery of sexual performance (strong erections, orgasmic ability) over intimacy and connection, even though in the real world both women and men value intimacy from partner sex. It is also clear that the idealized version of sex only focuses on a tiny sliver of sexuality—vaginal intercourse—even though men's and women's sexual lives are far more varied and rich than this implies.

The ideal model of sex (some aspects of which have been termed the "fantasy model" of sex by Bernie Zilbergeld, PhD, author of *The New Male Sexuality*) is reflected in how women and men talk to their friends about sex. For instance, when girl-friends ask one another if a new boyfriend is "good in bed," they usually mean—is he "good" at intercourse. More specifically, does he last long enough and can he "give" the woman an orgasm. Even if a woman really enjoys oral sex, mutual mastur-bation, toy play, or breast play, this stereotypical conversation focuses solely on vaginal intercourse, as if that were the only way to evaluate sexual satisfaction.

Of course, much of the sex that people actually enjoy doesn't resemble these ideals. For some women, their best sex has been with a man who ejaculated very quickly, thus leaving the woman wanting more, rather than wishing sex would end. A partner who is bound and determined to give a woman an orgasm during intercourse would perhaps leave a woman feeling pressured if she wasn't very interested in having an orgasm at all, or frustrated if she preferred to have them another way and he wouldn't listen. Some men and women are enormously turned on by extensive vaginal wetness or female ejaculation; others prefer sex that is drier. But no matter what your ideal preferences are, many people find that erections, orgasms, and lubrication matter far less than feeling comfortable with and connected to a partner. That's because in the real world, sex that feels relaxed, pleasurable, playful, and intimate feels better than sex that is based on chasing down performance goals.

HOMEWORK
Mirror Play

This exercise can be done by yourself or with a partner. It requires comfort, a willingness to be silly, and trust in one another.

If you're trying this exercise with a partner, begin by getting naked in front of a mirror (the bigger the better) and remarking how your bodies are similar to or different from each other (this is more fun than it may sound and can feel quite silly)—from your hips to your chests to your genitals and your feet, and from both the front and back. (Kneel or get on all fours, turn around, and then crane your heads to see your backsides.) Bend over to look at your butts from different angles. Remember, too, that you are each other's caretakers—most people have some sensitivities related to their bodies, and you will need to be thoughtful, gentle, and kind in terms of the similarities and differences that you note. That said, do try to let yourselves go and to laugh and enjoy this exercise. When else have you had the chance—let alone when has anyone else urged you—to play "I'll show you mine if you show me yours" as an adult?

If you're trying this exercise by yourself, try looking at your body in a mirror not from a critical perspective, but with interest, curiosity, and enjoyment. Note your curves and how they feel to your touch. (Softness is a very sensual and desirable characteristic.) Check out your breasts and how they've changed over time, and remember: This isn't a bad thing. Having age-appropriate expectations of your body is a desire-enhancer. Make sure to pay special attention to the parts of you that a previous or present partner has admired, or that you have always particularly liked or found sexy.

Your Vagina Tents!

*Lessons That Can Change
Your Sex Life for the Better*

For many women, sexual desire and arousal may seem like
the same thing. But technically, they are different processes.
Desire is a term generally used to describe feelings of sexual
interest, whereas arousal refers to the sexually excited state of
both mind and body. When a woman is young, first beginning
her sex life, or when she is in a new relationship, desire and
arousal may feel particularly interchangeable—and relatively
effortless. The high hormone levels of youth and the chemical
changes associated with falling in love (or lust) can spark
frequent feelings of sexual arousal and desire. It can be difficult to tease apart the differences between the two when you are
frequently in the mood—and ready—to be sexual with a partner.

Because desire and arousal are often experienced simultaneously, at least at the beginning of a sexual relationship or during a brief fling, women sometimes become accustomed to relying on their bodies for cues to when they want to have sex. You may, for example, have had the experience of feeling a tingling or warmth in your genitals and then realized that you must be feeling aroused or full of desire. Sometimes women notice vaginal wetness (lubrication) or throbbing and interpret it as a sign of sexual interest. These can be enjoyable bodily sensations and "signs" of excitement and yet, as a relationship progresses or as a woman ages, her body may take longer to respond or she may not notice these signs as easily, as often, or as strongly as she once did. This can make some women wonder what has happened to their experience of arousal and excitement.

In this chapter, we'll advance our conversation about desire and delve more deeply into issues of arousal, which, like many sexual issues, involves both mind and body. But first, some questions for you.

POP QUIZ

1. Which of these generally occur during sexual excitement and arousal?

    a. Increase in heart rate

    b. Increase in vaginal lubrication

    c. Increase in bloodflow to the genitals

    d. Increase in vaginal size

    e. All of the above

2. In the United States, roughly what percentage of women experience problems with lubrication?

    a. 10%

    b. 21%

    c. 31%

    d. 45%

3. Personal lubricants can do all of the following *except:*

    a. Prevent sexually transmissible diseases (STDs)

    b. Help sex feel more comfortable

    c. Help sex feel more pleasurable

    d. Reduce the risk of tearing during intercourse

4. Silicone-based lubricant can safely be used by women who are using all of the following forms of contraception *except:*

    a. Birth control pill

    b. Silicone diaphragm

    c. Condom

    d. All of the above

Answers: 1) e; 2) c; 3) a; 4) b

    The fact that nearly one-third of women experience lubrication problems (based on findings from a scientific survey of 987 women in the United States)[1] surprises many people—mostly because women and men tend to think of lubrication difficulties as something experienced by women who are older or postmenopausal. And yet many women—even those in their twenties, thirties, and forties—find that natural vaginal lubrication doesn't always come easily or that the amount of lubrication that a woman's body produces may not be sufficient for comfortable or pleasurable sex. Even when women feel emotionally aroused or interested in sex, their physical body doesn't always respond with sufficient vaginal lubrication or other signs of arousal. Because talking about sex remains taboo in many cultures, many women don't know that this is a common experience shared by women of various ages. As a result, women may feel frustrated and confused about why sex feels uncomfortable even when they want to have it, or why they need to use a lubricant in order to have satisfying sex.

I want to create for you a safe, no-taboo zone in which we can talk openly about sexual arousal and lubrication. As such, I have the following goals for you in this chapter. I'd like for you to:

* Learn more about some of the truly fascinating things that occur in your body during arousal and how you can apply this knowledge to create more comfortable, pleasurable sex

* Identify at least two strategies you can use to attend to or increase your own sexual arousal

* Be able to rewrite your own story to promote your sexual arousal

* Understand how lifestyle and health-related choices can affect sexual arousal

* Feel comfortable talking with your partner (if you have one) about what enhances your arousal and about how both of your bodies respond to sexual excitement and arousal

WHAT EXACTLY IS AROUSAL, ANYWAY?

Sexual arousal is an integral part of sexual response. Sometimes a woman feels aroused first, before any sexual activity takes place; other times, a woman might get into foreplay or sex and then, over time, notice that she develops feelings of arousal, excitement, and feeling "into it." Some women find that even if they don't feel 100 percent up to it at first, once they start to have sex, they think, "Wow, this feels good! How come we don't do this more often?" For a lot of women, arousal can take a few minutes to kick in before they experience the physical and mental effects of feeling warm, tingly, well lubricated (wet), and turned-on.

In fact, our bodies undergo many changes during sexual arousal and excitement, and some of these changes take time. Our heart rate increases, breathing quickens, and bloodflow increases to the genitals, resulting in greater vaginal lubrication and a feeling of pressure or fullness in or around the vagina. You may feel some sensation in or around the clitoris (which enlarges slightly) and vagina. Some women even report feeling particularly intense sensations—even throbbing—along the front wall of their vagina (the G-spot area), which may occur due to the swelling of the internal parts of the clitoris or the overall pressure that results from increased bloodflow. Many women also describe feeling warm in their genitals, or feeling as though they have to pee even if they've recently emptied their bladder. (Again, this may be related to the urethra's close proximity to and interconnection with the clitoris and vagina—a change to one may affect sensation in the others.) In addition, muscular tension builds throughout the body via a process called **myotonia**, which may result in involuntary curling of your lips or toes, or a stiffening of your legs as excitement builds. Even our breasts undergo physical changes—they enlarge slightly, and the nipples often become erect.

Vaginal Tenting (My Favorite Arousal Response)

One of the most fascinating changes related to sexual arousal (at least as far as I'm concerned) is called vaginal tenting. Here is what happens: Although a woman's vaginal canal is 3 to 4 inches long when she is unaroused, as she becomes sexually aroused, muscular tension pulls the uterus upward, which creates more space inside the vagina. This is sometimes described as the vagina "growing" or "expanding" in both length and width, notably in the inner two-thirds of the vagina. The vagina that starts out 3 to 4 inches long becomes at least 6 inches long, in many cases. (Which, not coincidentally, is enough room to comfortably accommodate the average-size penis.)

It's important to understand this process of vaginal tenting and the ways in which excitement encourages vaginal lubrication, as it may help you figure out how to make sex feel more comfortable and pleasurable. If you experience any of the following situations, you may find it helpful to spend extra time in foreplay to encourage your arousal response.

* It feels like your partner uncomfortably hits up against your cervix during vaginal intercourse.

* Your partner's penis is especially long or wide.

* You experience uncomfortable vaginal dryness during penetration.

* You're prone to tiny cuts or tears during intercourse.

In addition to increasing your physical comfort, spending more time in foreplay can also increase pleasure. Some women find that waiting to begin intercourse until they are highly aroused, lubricated, and throbbing with excitement results in more pleasurable intercourse, a more (enjoyably) sensitive vagina, and more potential for orgasm—or even multiple orgasm.

I cannot emphasize enough how important it is for couples to understand female sexual arousal so that they can create a more satisfying and mutually enjoyable sex life. Several years ago, a young woman came to me for help. She and her boyfriend had been dating for 2 years and were very much in love, but they simply could not find a way to have comfortable sex. No matter what they tried, intercourse was painful for her. They attributed this to her boyfriend's larger-than-average penis size. They saw this problem as impossible to fix and worried that they would have to end their otherwise happy relationship.

I described how spending more time in foreplay and doing things that felt exciting to her could encourage her arousal response, which would result in increased vaginal lubrication (to facilitate comfortable penetration) and more space in her vagina, thanks to vaginal tenting (which was needed for sex with her above-average-size boyfriend). I suggested, too, that they keep a store-bought lubricant near the bed in case her natural vaginal lubrication wasn't sufficient for his size, even after extended foreplay. The next week, she reported back to me that for the first time in their 2-year relationship, they'd had comfortable, pleasurable, and extremely arousing sex. And while they were happy about having better sex, they were thrilled that their relationship didn't have to end. To this day, their story still touches me. We all want to find someone to spend our days and nights with, someone whom we not only love (and who loves us back), but with whom we can live, and it's heartbreaking to think that this couple nearly split over something that—with a little bit of education about arousal and lubrication—was entirely fixable.

Female Sexual Arousal Disorder: Differences Matter

For some couples, information and education are all it takes to improve sex. However, some sexual problems are more complex and may be influenced by medical conditions, long-standing relationship problems, issues of trust, communication problems, or past traumas (such as sexual abuse or assault). Just as women's lives are varied, so are their sexual problems. For many years, women who struggled with sexual arousal were treated as if they were all the same. Research conducted in the past decade, however, suggests that there may be different subcategories of women who experience Female Sexual Arousal Disorder (SAD), including those that may be described as having Genital SAD, Subjective SAD, or Combined SAD. In addition, there are practical reasons why these differences may matter in terms of causes and treatment.

Women with Genital SAD may have no problem feeling aroused mentally, but their bodies don't seem to respond. Regardless of age, women with Genital SAD may feel as though their vaginal lubrication is low and not sufficient for comfortable intercourse, and they aren't able to experience pleasant genital sensations even when they feel psychologically aroused. Women who have been diagnosed with certain medical problems (such as diabetes or hypertension) may be particularly prone to impaired physical arousal.

Women with Subjective SAD, on the other hand, may experience all of the typical bodily changes one would expect

●

during arousal, including increases in vaginal lubrication and feelings of vaginal warmth, tingling, or fullness, and yet they don't feel mentally or emotionally aroused. Some women who experience Subjective SAD may say that they feel like their bodies are revved up and ready to go, but they themselves don't feel engaged, excited, or "into it." They may wonder what it means that they don't, in their minds and hearts, feel aroused by their partner. And yet a lack of mental arousal isn't necessarily a sign of a relationship problem. In fact, women may find that—with practice—they can teach themselves how to notice their sexually responsive bodies and recognize such signs as related to positive feelings of arousal or excitement.

The third subgroup, those with Combined SAD, may feel a broader range of difficulty with arousal, in the sense that they neither feel genitally aroused (warm, tingly, lubricated) nor psychologically aroused. Women who fall into any of these three categories may feel confused by their sexual arousal response (or lack of it), frustrated by it, and unsure how to address it privately or together with their partner. In addition, women who experience arousal problems may also experience other sexual difficulties. For example, many women who experience low arousal may also find it difficult to experience desire. (You can imagine how women with low lubrication due to arousal problems might find sex uncomfortable and then eventually come to desire sex less often, thus creating a cycle.) Other times, women with arousal problems may find it difficult to orgasm. After all, if a woman doesn't find herself physically or emotionally aroused in the first place, it can be difficult for her to reach a point where she feels so intensely excited that she is able to orgasm.

At this writing, only a small amount of research has been

conducted on subtypes of sexual arousal disorder, and we are still learning more about which treatments (including counseling, prescription medications, over-the-counter supplements, and lifestyle changes) may be particularly helpful to women in each subgroup. If you are experiencing low desire, I would encourage you to read through this chapter to learn about some of the strategies that have worked for other women who have faced these challenges, and then consider what you might try comfortably. You may also consider meeting with a trained sex therapist (see Resources on page 234) who can help you identify personalized strategies.

THE IMPORTANCE OF STORYTELLING

Several years ago I was sitting with Julia Heiman, PhD, in her office at the Kinsey Institute. She had recently become director of the Institute following many years at the University of Washington (UW), and I had made an appointment with her to discuss my research interests, learn about hers, and get to know her. At one point she mentioned that one of her research interests related to how people change. To illustrate this, she told me about a research study that she and another psychologist, Stephanie Kuffel, PhD, PS, a clinical assistant professor with the University of Washington Medical School, had recently completed.[2]

Dr. Heiman and Dr. Kuffel recruited women (some of whom had symptoms of mild depression) to come to a research lab, complete questionnaires, and listen to a very brief recording (about 30 seconds long) that asked them to adopt or "try on" two different sexual personas: either that of a woman who initiated and enjoyed sex and its physical sensations (including orgasm), or that of a woman who felt sex was not important or enjoyable and that orgasms were not satisfying. These recordings were essentially opposites—for example, the positive recording began with the phrases "You like your sexuality a lot. Sex is a very important part of your life . . ." and the negative recording began with "You do not like your sexuality. Sex is not very important in your life . . ."

These women were not given medication or treatment of any kind, other than an audio recording of the identity that they were asked to "try on" prior to watching a sexually explicit film clip while in a private space. (Asking women and men to watch erotic clips while their physical responses are monitored privately with lab equipment is a common technique used in sexuality research.)

Dr. Heiman and Dr. Kuffel found that after taking on the "positive" identity, women in the study not only *reported* higher levels of arousal while watching the film (compared to when they were asked to take on the "negative" identity), but their bodies also showed physical signs of arousal. Specifically, when women assumed the positive identity, the pattern of bloodflow to their genitals increased as compared to when they assumed the negative identity. The positive story seemed to encourage higher levels of arousal in both mental and physical sexual response.

Of course, this doesn't mean that if we tell ourselves positive short stories about our sexuality that we can sustain changes in our sexual response over a period of time. We might be able to— but we need more research to understand how long the effects of such stories would last on a person or how often she might need to repeat such stories to create lasting change. In fact, asking patients to reframe the way they think about themselves and to change the stories they tell themselves is a common technique in many forms of therapy—sexual or otherwise. You might recognize this as an "Act as if" strategy (such as "Act as if you're confident, even if you're not").

That said, the results of this study suggest that in spite of the race to develop sexual enhancement products for women (the so-called "female Viagra"), there is a great deal to learn about individual psychologies. We have the capacity to experience pleasure and greater levels of arousal—and to ultimately change our experience of sexuality—in ways that we may overlook or undervalue. Though medication is certainly helpful for many people, it's not the only option. We all have the capacity to invite pleasure into our lives, to "try on" the identity of a woman who likes and enjoys sex, and to learn what strategies work for each of us.

PAYING ATTENTION

The mind-body connection is particularly important when it comes to sexual arousal. Women's physical sexual arousal doesn't always line up with their emotional and mental experiences of arousal. For example, in sex research studies that take place in a laboratory, scientists find that it is not unusual for a woman to say that she did not feel sexually aroused by certain stimuli (such as an erotic film clip) even though the laboratory equipment measuring her body's physical response clearly showed that her body experienced an arousal response. Just because our bodies respond to arousal does not mean that we recognize or interpret these changes in ways that feel good or sexually exciting.

Some sex therapists, counselors, and educators have found

that women can improve their experience of sexual arousal by tuning in to their bodily sensations and responses, almost as a way of giving themselves "cues" or "feedback." For some women, paying special attention to these bodily responses can help to jump-start their mental arousal so that they feel more excited and "into" sex. Taking the time to notice whether you are experiencing any of these arousal responses can help you feel aroused, excited, or interested in sex (particularly if you apply the mindfulness exercise from page 185). These physical sensations may feel as though they are focused in or around your genitals (feelings of vaginal fullness, pulsing, warmth, or wetness), breasts (breast tenderness, nipple hardening), or somewhere else altogether (such as butterflies in your stomach). I've even heard from women who realize they're feeling aroused when their lip or toes start to curl involuntarily or when they start to feel jittery or excited. What's important is that, over time, you learn to identify your personal signs of arousal.

If you experience any of these sensations, take note of how you feel emotionally and mentally as you experience them. Do these sensations trigger feelings of excitement, pleasure, curiosity, or happiness? Or do they trigger feelings of discomfort, avoidance, shame, anxiety, or sadness? These feelings are worth paying attention to, as some arousal problems are rooted not in the body's inability to become aroused but rather in a negative interpretation of arousal. Women who have been abused or who have been made to feel ashamed of or guilty about their sexuality (or their bodies) may be particularly prone to such negative interpretations. If you find yourself responding negatively to your own arousal, consider ways in which you can challenge these critical voices in your head. If

•

you would like personalized guidance or support through this process, you might find it helpful to meet with a sex therapist.

IMPROVING AROUSAL

Given the different ways that women experience arousal, there are also numerous ways that women can inspire or enhance their physical or mental arousal. Below I've listed some tips that have been successful for many women. As you read through, consider which strategies you might want to try.

✱ **Attend to your emotions.** As important as it can be to notice and respond positively to physical sensations of arousal, paying attention to emotions is another way to promote sexual arousal. Even if you have had difficult or hurtful moments in your relationship (most people have), try to remember that couples have to start somewhere in their effort to reconnect. If you notice the slightest feelings of excitement, eagerness, connection, or joy in regard to how you feel about your partner or being sexual together, try to focus on those feelings and think about what it would be like to be physically intimate together, whether through holding hands, kissing, or being sexual in other ways.

✱ **Seek to understand your partner.** In a 2004 study,[3] women said that they found it easier to become (or stay) aroused if they felt that their partner liked or was attracted to their body, was involved with or concerned about family planning (such as choosing a birth control method), and accepted (or felt aroused by) their body's sexual response (in terms of their noises, moans, wetness, and orgasmic style). Unfortunately, many women have exactly this type

of preferred partner but—due to a lack of communication—
they may not realize it! Some women assume that because
their partner doesn't ask about birth control, he isn't
interested in their relationship; or they might think that
if he doesn't offer lots of compliments, he doesn't find
her sexy. If you have doubts or questions about how your
partner feels about you, or if you've assumed that your
partner's silence signals his discontent, try talking to
him in a way that promotes sharing and understanding.
It may make a difference in your feelings of acceptance,
love, and—ultimately—arousal.

✱ **Stretch your limits.** Sometimes women find that
stepping outside of their comfort zone, even just a bit,
can feel incredibly arousing. Try to identify two or
three things that you find very appealing in your
fantasy world. Can you imagine a scenario in which you
might feel comfortable being sexual in this way? For
example, if you are used to making love in the dark but
would like to pull your partner into the bedroom (or
pantry!) in the middle of the day, try to think of a way
to do this that feels comfortable and sexy. Is there a
type of lingerie you would like to wear, a sex position
you'd like to try, or some dirty words you'd like to
whisper in your partner's ear during sex? Trying
something new and daring can feel thrilling, exciting,
and—you guessed it—arousing. If you're looking for
ideas, you might browse women-friendly erotic stories
(see Resources on page 234).

✱ **Go for a run!** If you've ever felt physically aroused after a
workout, listen up: Several studies suggest that vigorous,
moderately timed exercise can increase women's genital

•

arousal responses.[4] To see how it works for you, try going on a vigorous run, walk, or bike ride for about 20 minutes, and then make note of your genital responses. Exercise's effects on sexual arousal tend to be strongest shortly after exercise, but you can take over where exercise leaves off by engaging in sex play privately or with a partner and encouraging your own sexual response. Think of exercise as a gentle boost in the direction of arousal.

✱ **De-stress.** For some women, sex brings up all kinds of anxieties: whether they will be good enough in bed, whether their partner finds them attractive, or whether their body will respond with pleasure or orgasm in the way that they want it to. Not only does stress feel unpleasant, but it can also interfere with sexual arousal. Some women find that slow, deep breaths can enhance their arousal, whereas others find that very deep but quick breathing patterns can enhance arousal (probably by activating the sympathetic nervous system, which is involved in sexual response). Try both breathing patterns to see which works best for you, and focus your mind on positive, relaxing thoughts.

✱ **Cut out the smoke.** As if you needed another reason to steer clear of cigarettes, research suggests that nicotine can impair a woman's sexual response.[5] In this study, nonsmoking women were asked to chew on nicotine gum or a placebo gum that looked, tasted, and smelled like the nicotine gum, and to watch an erotic film about 40 minutes later. The women who chewed the nicotine gum showed decreased genital arousal.

✳ **Relish foreplay.** Many women (and men, too!) wish they spent more time in foreplay, and for good reason—it encourages both women's and men's sexual responses. For women, foreplay encourages vaginal tenting and lubrication. For men, foreplay can make it easier to get and maintain an erection. Often, when two people have been together for a long time, they take their clothes off very quickly and jump into sex. Why not spend 10 to 20 minutes kissing with your clothes on as a way to enhance arousal prior to beginning intercourse? Both women and men often say that by building arousal they build sexual tension, too, which can make sexual play and penetration feel more seductive and pleasurable and can even make it easier for a woman to orgasm (sometimes multiple times). Some sex therapists recommend that couples hold out for as long as they can before starting intercourse—possibly even to the point where women feel as though their vagina is throbbing or pulsing with arousal. Try it and see how it feels for you.

✳ **Let go of anger.** Anger and blame are the enemies of arousal. If you are mad, whether with yourself or at your partner, those feelings need to be addressed outside of the bedroom. It can feel heavy and burdensome to carry anger and negativity, and it can be a great relief to forgive, reconcile, speak your mind, or let go, as the case may be. Negative feelings can create big barriers in intimate relationships.

✳ **Self-pleasure.** Some women find that they prefer to practice improving their sexual arousal when they are in private, during self-pleasuring. Using a lubricant to self-pleasure with one's fingers or a sex toy can feel more pleasurable (and potentially more arousing) than sexual play without a lubricant, although either method feels great for many women. Preliminary research suggests that an arousal fluid, Zestra, which is available over the counter in many drug stores, may help to increase women's sexual arousal, too.[6]

* **Talk to your doctor.** Although many cases of arousal problems are best addressed in sex therapy or with one's partner, there are cases in which arousal problems may be a sign of a medical condition or where medical treatment may help to enhance a woman's arousal responses. For example, women with diabetes and hypertension are more vulnerable to experiencing low arousal. Similarly, women who are taking certain antidepressants may experience a range of sexual side effects, including impaired arousal. Other times, a healthcare provider may suggest lifestyle changes, such as increased exercise or nutritional adjustments.

LUBRICANTS

Although vaginal lubrication is an important part of sexual arousal for many women, some sexual health professionals worry that too much has been made of the connection between lubrication and arousal—almost to the point where some women have been described as having an "arousal disorder" when they simply don't lubricate as much as they might like to. Feelings of vaginal dryness may be caused by or associated with a number of factors, though, including little time spent in foreplay, menopause, or side effects from hormonal medications (including low-estrogen birth control pills). Women may also feel particularly dry if they try to have sex shortly after taking a warm bath or shower or after swimming, as water can wash away natural lubrication and cause them to feel dry. In other instances, a woman may produce a substantial amount of vaginal lubrication, but if her partner's penis is particularly large or if sex lasts for a very long time, she may feel as though she needs additional lubrication in order to have comfortable, pleasurable sex. Most women and men in the United States (about 70 percent) have used a personal lubricant during sex, and there is nothing wrong with or unusual about trying one.

The three most common lubricant types are water-based, silicone-based, and oil-based. **Water-based lubricants** are the most commonly sold and are often described as feeling natural or more similar to vaginal lubrication. Because they are water-based, however, they absorb easily into women's and men's bodies, which may mean that couples will want to reapply lubricant if sex lasts for a long time or begins to feel uncomfortable. **Silicone-based lubricants** tend to feel slick compared to other types. Because they last longer than water-based lubricants, they are often preferred for marathon sex or masturbation sessions. Also, silicone-based lubricants won't wash away easily with water, so they are better suited for sex that takes place in the shower, bath, or hot tub. One consideration, however, is that silicone lubricants should not be used in conjunction with other silicone products, such as a silicone diaphragm or silicone sex toy, as the combination can be abrasive to the diaphragm or toy. **Oil-based lubricants** should not be used with latex condoms, as they can cause latex to break or tear. This includes olive oil, which is sometimes recommended by

●

gynecologists as a natural lubricant but is generally not considered safe to use with latex. If you need to use condoms but you prefer an oil-based lubricant, consider using a polyurethane condom with your lubricant.

Although some women and men use **saliva** as a lubricant, this practice is generally not recommended—particularly for women who are prone to yeast infections. Using saliva as a lubricant for vaginal intercourse can increase some women's chances of getting yeast infections, as can cunnilingus (oral sex performed on a woman). This is mostly true for women who are prone to frequent yeast infections; other women often enjoy these activities without ever developing a yeast infection. If you're vulnerable to repeated yeast infections, you might ask your partner to take a shower before having sex or to wash his penis with a warm, damp cloth before sex. (I know it doesn't sound sexy, but I'm convinced that with enough creativity, a woman can make just about *anything* seem sexy.) If you perform oral sex on him before vaginal sex, dab his penis with the warm, damp cloth after fellatio but before vaginal sex. And if you enjoy cunnilingus but don't want to get a yeast infection, try using a latex dental dam or a condom cut in half lengthwise as a barrier between your vulva and his mouth.

Finally, keep in mind that **lotions** and **creams** are not lubricants. These types of products may be damaging to latex condoms (increasing their risk of breakage) and may also cause vaginal irritation or sensitivity. Instead, stick to products that are specifically made for sexual activity. More details about choosing lubricants to use with sex toys or when considering certain sexual health concerns or fertility-related issues are included in Chapters 7 and 8.

•

FACT: *Sometimes lubricant is not enough.*

Although personal lubricants can make sex more comfortable and pleasurable for many women, some women have genital pain conditions that require more than the use of a lubricant. If you have had painful sex in spite of spending more time in foreplay, using a lubricant, or trying more comfortable sex positions, I would strongly encourage you to see a medical professional who has expertise in issues related to vulvar pain conditions, such as vulvodynia. (See page 35 for related information and resources.)

MYTH: *Men are the only visual creatures.*

Although men are commonly described as being more "visual" than women, we know that many women experience sexual arousal as a result of watching erotic films and videos, too. Women, however, are often more aroused by films and videos that have been made by other women. These films tend to include more foreplay and context for the sexual relationship, whereas male-oriented films tend to focus on penetration and close-up shots of women's and men's genitals. If you're interested in learning about porn and erotica made by women, look for titles by Candida Royalle, Estelle Joseph, and Annie Sprinkle, for starters. Women's sex boutiques often carry a wide range of titles, too.

Using a Lubricant: The Basics

Who applies the lubricant? Either partner! You may find that you're more turned on either by applying it to your partner's genitals or to your own body, or from watching your partner lube one (or both of you) up.

How much should I use? Less is more in the case of lube. (If you use too much, you may feel less sensation during intercourse.) Start out with a dime-size amount and then use less or more as you see fit.

•

HOMEWORK
Writing Your Story

Keeping in mind that the stories we tell ourselves can change our physical and emotional experiences of sex, can you imagine a story that might help to encourage your arousal? Your story doesn't have to be long, it just has to make sense to you and be something that you can think about when you are trying to expand your arousal and approach pleasure with an open mind. Yours might look like one of these.

"I love my husband, and I find him so sexy. I can't wait to be with him, and to have him touch me, kiss me, hold me, and love me."

"I love having sex, getting off, being naked, and feeling wet and warm."

"Sex is fun, invigorating, and gets me going."

"Having sex helps me to feel free and like I can let go. I like the way that my breasts tingle, and how I feel wet and lubricated, and as though we simply cannot get enough of each other."

Sometimes women find it easier to write themselves a new sex-positive story if they first consider the negative stories that they are

---

Where should we apply the lubricant? It can be applied to your genitals, your partner's genitals, the sex toy that you're using, or to either of your fingers (and then to either of your genitals). In the case of vaginal intercourse, some couples only apply it to one partner, whereas others apply lubricant to both partners' genitals. Experiment and see what feels most arousing and pleasurable to you.

How do you use a lubricant with condoms? Applying a small dab (about the size of one or two peas) in the inside tip of a already telling themselves. For example, one woman told me that most of her sex had become "duty sex"—sex that she gave in and had with her husband out of a sense of obligation rather than pleasure. They had two young children and she said that, at the end of a long, tiring, day, she would dread sex, thinking, "Here we go again, he's going to paw my breasts until I give in. He doesn't even care about what my day's been like." No one would want to have sex if that was the story playing in their mind! This woman loved her husband and found him attractive, but rarely felt excited about having sex with him. Together, we imagined other stories that she could tell herself that might change her experience. Using her negative story as a starting place, we turned the negatives into positives, which resulted in a new story that she could tell herself: "My husband is so crazy in love with me, and so turned on by my body, that he can barely contain himself." Telling herself this new story, in combination with learning to reject his advances with kindness (see Chapter 1) on nights when she truly did not have the energy to have sex, formed a new strategy for embracing feel-good sex.

condom can make intercourse pleasurable for your male partner. Don't apply too much, however, or it could cause the condom to slip off. Feel free to apply slightly more lubricant on the outside of the condom after it is already on the penis. If you're concerned about condom slippage, make sure to check every now and then to make sure that the condom is still on. Also, your male partner should always hold on to the base of the condom when he is withdrawing his penis from your body, regardless of whether or not you are using lubricant.

The Optional Orgasm

*Take the Pressure Off
and Let the Pleasure In*

Whether you find it easy or difficult to orgasm, believe that orgasms are vital to your sex life, or see them as simply an over-hyped phenomenon, most of us want to learn more about this elusive sensation. And for good reason! Orgasms, in some sense, are everywhere—regardless of whether or not they're in our bedrooms. We read about them in magazines, hear about them from friends, and may feel excited (or pressured) to experience them with a partner.

Even if you think you have it all figured out, your experience with orgasms is likely to change over the years as you age and experience life or relationship changes. Orgasms can also be influenced by physical and hormonal changes. You may find that certain positions or sex acts feel more or less pleasurable while pregnant, or that orgasms become easier or more difficult to experience in the months after giving birth. Your orgasmic response can also be influenced by hormonal contraception, menopause, or a hysterectomy.

Other times, orgasm changes may have nothing to do with your body and everything to do with your partner, your relationship, or your personal growth. Maybe you have a new partner who, unlike your ex, has a strong desire to stimulate you to orgasm, which makes you want to identify your orgasm triggers. Or maybe your current partner is more supportive than previous partners of the fact that reaching orgasm is less interesting to you than exploring other pleasurable ways of enjoying sexual intimacy. Or your partner and relationship may stay the same, but you may change. You may grow in terms of your confidence or knowledge of your body or your willingness to experiment sexually, or you may become more curious about and committed to sexual intimacy in a way that affects your orgasmic or pleasure-focused response.

We all have different expectations about and desires for our personal experiences of sexual pleasure and orgasm. My role is not to suggest which choices are right for you but simply to provide information that will help you to feel comfortable and confident about your options for having sex that feels good. Whether you want to focus on pleasure, have more regular orgasms, or bring your orgasms back from who-knows-where-they've-been, there is something in this chapter for you. First: our quiz.

POP QUIZ

1. Approximately what percentage of women orgasm rarely, or never, during intercourse?

    a. 5%
    b. 15%
    c. 20%
    d. 33%

2. Which one of the factors below has been shown to be strongly associated with more pleasurable and satisfying orgasms for women?

    a. G-spot stimulation
    b. Clitoral stimulation
    c. Psychological intensity of the sexual experience
    d. Relationship satisfaction
    e. C and D only

3. Roughly how many *men* report that they have faked an orgasm?

    a. 10%
    b. 25%
    c. 40%
    d. 50%

4. At the time of an orgasm, a woman's body releases a large amount of a chemical called prolactin, which may make her:

    a. Feel satisfied
    b. Feel hungry
    c. Cry
    d. A and C only
    e. None of the above

5. Women are more likely to be more orgasmic when they are in relationships in which they and their partner can communicate about:

    a. Sexual acts that involve direct clitoral stimulation

    b. A range of sexual topics

    c. Her sexual fantasies

    d. Masturbation

Answers: 1) d; 2) e; 3) b; 4) d; 5) a

Well, what did you learn? My hope is that whether you've had zero orgasms or ten thousand orgasms, you will be curious enough to keep reading and learning about them—not just today, but throughout your life. Why? Because curiosity is fundamentally linked to good sex. Being curious can inspire you to learn more about your body and mind, including how they respond to and experience pleasure. Curiosity might also motivate you to learn more about your *partner's* body, desires, fantasies, and responses.

What would you like to know more about—what an orgasm feels like? What happens in our bodies, chemically speaking, during an orgasm? Whether different types of orgasms exist or feel better than other types? What enhances a woman's ability to orgasm alone or with a partner? If you're curious about any of these topics, you're like many other women and men—and you're in luck, as you're about to learn about all of the above.

Achieving orgasm isn't just about bodies, positions, or techniques. As shown in the quiz, studies suggest that the pleasure and satisfaction that come from an orgasm are more closely tied to a person's *psychological* experience—the feelings and thoughts they have related to a sexual encounter—than with the physical sensations, like which body parts were stimulated or how it felt (such as throbbing, pulsating, warm, tingly, and so on).

As such, although tips and techniques have a place in pleasure (and this chapter), so does our psychological experience. In fact, if you generally feel like you know your way around your own and your partner's body, but you would like to ramp up your pleasure potential, the missing puzzle piece may very well rest between your ears, rather than between your legs. Our minds are rich sources of fantasy, excitement, confidence, and knowledge—all of which can enrich our sexual lives. After reading and thinking about the information in this chapter, I believe that you will be better able to:

✳ Understand why orgasms feel pleasurable and satisfying for many women

✳ Feel that although an orgasm is one of many good things that can come of sex, there shouldn't be any pressure to "attain" one

✳ Identify at least two strategies that you can use to enhance your capacity for pleasure or achieving orgasm

✳ Communicate comfortably with a partner or close friend about your experiences, challenges, or curiosities related to sexual pleasure or orgasms

✳ Talk with a healthcare provider or counselor/therapist if you have questions about changes or difficulties related to your experience of sexual sensation, pleasure, or experiencing orgasm

WHAT IS AN ORGASM?

In my work as a sex educator and columnist, numerous women (and men) have asked what an orgasm feels like for a woman and how to tell if they (or their partner) have had one. Simply put, an orgasm is a brief climax (usually lasting fewer than 20 or 30 seconds) that results from the escalation of a woman's heart rate, breathing, body temperature, and muscular tension—all of which peak, and then release, at the time of orgasm. As an orgasm begins, women may become aware of a quick series of vaginal, uterine, and anal contractions. But that's not all—for many women, orgasm is a peak of pleasure, both emotionally and physically. Frequently, women describe intense feelings of ecstasy, wild abandon, euphoria, or calm ease that occur at the moment of orgasm and possibly for several (or many) minutes afterward. A woman may even shed a few tears after an orgasm. Some researchers speculate that orgasm-related tears result from the intense positive emotions experienced at orgasm; others suggest that such tears are the result of the hormone prolactin (more on this below), which is released in large amounts at the time of orgasm and has been linked to crying.

In many cases, an orgasm feels like a definite "event," thanks to the peak of physical sensations, which is perhaps why many women tell their orgasm-curious friends, "When you have one, you'll know it." Unlike sexual arousal and excitement, which may ebb and flow more subtly, orgasms tend to feel a little more "defined" for many women. That said, because women's bodies and psychological experiences vary, some women may have milder experiences of orgasm, which can make it tricky for them to figure out the difference between intense arousal and orgasm.

As for the anatomy of an orgasm—precisely what triggers it and how it works—we quite honestly don't know all the answers. We still have much to learn about both women's and men's orgasms. However, researchers have learned a bit about the chemical changes that occur in our bodies related to sexual excitement and orgasms. For example, on page 103 I mentioned a chemical called **prolactin**, which is released in large amounts at the time of both women's and men's orgasms and seems to be related to feelings of contentment and satiation. Recent research even suggests that women and men both may release larger amounts of prolactin during orgasms that occur through vaginal intercourse compared to orgasms that occur during other sexual activities.[1] Another chemical, **oxytocin,** is released during close touching, kissing, breast stimulation, and sexual excitement, and it reaches particularly high levels shortly after a woman reaches orgasm. Oxytocin gets quite a lot of play in mainstream media, as it is often associated with feelings of closeness and bonding and, as such, has occasionally been referred to as the "cuddle hormone." Studies suggest that it may also promote sleep[2]— which may be one of the reasons why you or your partner drift off shortly after having sex.

Either or both of these chemical changes may contribute to reasons why some (but not all) women describe intercourse-related orgasms as feeling more emotionally satisfying than other orgasms. That said, some people suspect that intercourse-related orgasms may feel more satisfying simply because during intercourse, a couple typically gets to bond and feel close in various ways—including kissing, touching, and whispering in each other's ears—that one cannot do, for example, during oral sex or certain other sexual activities.

ORGASM TYPES

Rumors about orgasms are almost as rampant as rumors about celebrities—and there is a lot of misinformation out there about types of orgasms. As a result, some women feel as though they should be able to have every type of orgasm imaginable or that something is wrong with them if they don't orgasm during intercourse. Similarly, some men feel inadequate, or as if they aren't good enough lovers, if their female partners don't orgasm at all or in the way that they expect or have seen in the movies. A quick history lesson may help to explain some of the forces that have shaped women's and men's perceptions of orgasms.

In 1933, Dr. Sigmund Freud suggested that the **clitoral orgasm** was part of a pattern seen among less "mature" women.[3] Conversely, he identified **vaginal orgasms** as a sign of mature development. However, interview data published in 1953 by Alfred Kinsey, ScD, and his colleagues in their groundbreaking book, *Sexual Behavior in the Human Female*, suggested that clitoral stimulation was key to many women's experiences of pleasure and orgasm.[4] This idea was later confirmed in the laboratory by William Masters, MD, and Virginia Johnson, who conducted important work in the field of human sexuality in the 1960s and 1970s. The vaginal versus clitoral debate took a new turn in the 1970s, when it was proposed that perhaps there were actually three types of orgasms: **vulval orgasms** (vaginal contractions that resulted from either clitoral or vaginal stimulation), **uterine orgasms** (usually resulting from penile stimulation of the cervix, with no vaginal contractions but with some amount of irregular breathing), and **blended orgasms** (a combination of vulval and uterine types). However, these descriptions of orgasm types were based on very limited data and contemporary researchers tend not to describe orgasms in these terms.

Enter the G-spot, which was popularized by the 1982 book *The G Spot* by Alice Kahn Ladas, MSS, EdD; Beverly Whipple, PhD; and John D. Perry, PhD.[5] These researchers named the G-spot after Dr. Ernst Grafenberg, a doctor who, in 1950, suggested that an area on the anterior (front) wall of the vagina was erotically sensitive for some women. The authors of the book were very careful to point out that although many women enjoy or orgasm from G-spot stimulation, and some may even experience female ejaculation, not all women do. They advised that enjoyment or orgasm from G-spot stimulation was no better or worse than clitoral stimulation or other forms of sexual pleasuring. This was important information because at the time of the book's publication, much of the focus in sexual literature had been on the clitoris as the center of women's sexual experience and orgasm. As such, women who experienced pleasure and orgasms from vaginal stimulation may have been left feeling inadequate. Yet no one was able to contain the media hype over the so-called G-spot. As such, **G-spot orgasms**

The G-Shot

In the past few years, some physicians have begun offering women the G-Shot—an injection of collagen into the front wall of a woman's vagina (G-spot area). Though some describe the injection as helping to promote a woman's "awareness" of her G-spot and others describe the potential for sexual enhancement or orgasm, at the time of this writing there have not been any published scientific studies on the advantages (or risks) of such an injection—or whether it even works! Talk to your doctor before making the decision to receive such a shot.

became yet another benchmark that some women feel pressured to achieve—with quite a few women still, to this day, feeling unhappy if they have not done so.

But are there really different types of orgasms, or are these distinctions more rumor that fact? Certainly it is common for women to say that orgasms feel different during intercourse than they do when achieved through other types of stimulation, or as Germaine Greer said in her 1970 book *The Female Eunuch*, "At all events a clitoral orgasm with a full [vagina] is nicer than a clitoral orgasm with an empty one, as far as I can tell at least."[6] In fact, some contemporary research suggests that a woman's body may release more prolactin during orgasms that occur though intercourse than during orgasms that result from other types of sexual stimulation. And other studies suggest that different types of muscular activity may be involved in orgasms resulting from stimulation of the anterior vaginal wall (G-spot area) compared to orgasms resulting from direct stimulation of the glans clitoris. This may explain why—for some women—so-called "G-spot orgasms" feel different than so-called "clitoral orgasms." Some women describe G-spot orgasms as feeling more intense and "wavelike" than clitoral orgasms, which are often described as powerful, sharp, or electric.

One challenging aspect of sorting orgasms into different categories is that there is a good deal of overlap in how orgasms occur. For example, even though it is common for people to talk about orgasms that result from clitoral stimulation, recent, cutting-edge research suggests that the vast majority of all orgasms likely involve the clitoris (or, as it is increasingly called, "the clitoral complex"—the interconnected network of various parts of the clitoris, vagina, and urethra).[7] So if G-spot orgasms involve the clitoris, and if the clitoral parts swell during other types of sexual stimulation, such as breast play or mental fantasy, then aren't all orgasms, in essence, clitoral (or, at the very least, blended) orgasms?

We certainly know that women may reach orgasm from a wide range of activities, such as direct stimulation of the glans clitoris, the anterior wall of the vagina (G-spot), the back wall of the vagina, the cervix, the breasts, and even (for a small minority of women) from mental fantasy alone, without any physical touching whatsoever. Women, like men, sometimes even experience an orgasm during sleep.

My take on the orgasm-type debate is this: With more research, we may find that there are indeed several distinct types of female orgasms, but at the moment there isn't enough evidence to draw any hard conclusions. What we do know is that women may experience an orgasm from various types of stimulation and that not all women experience orgasms at all, let alone from each type of stimulation. I encourage any woman who wants to learn more about her potential for orgasms and

Faking It

Most women—and about one-quarter of men—say that they've pretended to have an orgasm when they didn't really have one. Often, they do so for similar reasons, including wanting to make their partner feel good, wanting to end sex, or feeling insecure that they were not able to orgasm even though they wanted to. Instead of brushing up on your acting skills, try being more open and genuine with your partner about your physical experience—you don't have to have an orgasm in order for it to be "good sex," and you shouldn't have to fake it in order to end it.

pleasure to explore her own body, without any expectations or pressures. As stated in Chapter 4, stress can make it very difficult to experience an orgasm. Try instead to focus on enjoyment, pleasure, and exploration when becoming familiar with your body and its sexual response.

LACK OF ORGASM

Although the vast majority of men report that they've experienced orgasms, fewer women do—either during masturbation or during sex with a partner. Orgasms aren't, as some people would suggest, "like riding a bike." It is not about learning a skill. Some women who have previously been orgasmic (even very easily or reliably orgasmic) may find that there are times in

Involve Your Partner!

Women sometimes feel embarrassed or inadequate if they have never had, or have difficulty experiencing, an orgasm. Research and clinical experience, however, consistently highlight that lack of female orgasm is often a couple issue, rather than something that is "wrong" with a woman. In some cases, a couple's communication has been linked to a woman's lack of orgasm, with such couples being more likely to blame each other and less likely to be receptive, attentive, and accepting of one another's viewpoints when talking about sex. Sex therapists commonly note the benefits of involving both partners in efforts to address a woman's lack of orgasm—and considering that several exercises related to facilitating women's orgasm involve sensual and sexual activities, involving one's partner can feel connecting, fun, and pleasurable, too.

●

their lives when it feels very difficult to orgasm, or times when orgasms don't feel as pleasurable or intense as they once did.

How common is it, then, to have difficulty experiencing an orgasm or to not experience one at all? A study of Americans conducted in the early 1990s reported that nearly a quarter of women—24 percent—had experienced a lack of orgasms (from either masturbation or partner sex) for at least several months during the previous year. Similar numbers have been found in other smaller studies and among women living in other countries. Even more women don't have orgasms during sex with a partner—specifically, one-third of women never, or only rarely (meaning less than 25 percent of the time), orgasm during intercourse with a partner. So, what gives?

WHO HAS ORGASMS AND WHO DOESN'T?

There are no hard-and-fast rules about what differentiates women who have orgasms from women who don't, although we are slowly discovering new pieces of the puzzle thanks to ongoing research in the area of female sexuality. It has long been known, for example, that women with higher levels of formal education may orgasm more frequently during masturbation compared to women with a high school education;[8] that said, there doesn't seem to be any relationship between education and whether or not a woman orgasms *with a partner*. Feeling guilty or negative about sex can also impair a woman's ability to have an orgasm as can certain health problems. For example, some research suggests that women who have Type 2 diabetes are more prone to orgasmic difficulties, as are some women with multiple sclerosis, perhaps due to changes in genital sensation.

LOVE, INTIMACY, AND ORGASM

A 2007 study found that the more women were in love with or felt emotionally close with their partner, the more they reported that orgasm was both satisfying and easy to attain; yet there was no correlation between their ratings of being in love and their *frequency* of achieving an orgasm.[9] Also, which comes first—the love or the ease of orgasm—is currently not known. It may be that women who feel more in love with or close to their partners have sex in different or more intimate, tender, or exciting ways than women who feel less in love with their partners. Perhaps they build arousal more intensely or, given their feelings of closeness, they may feel more comfortable relaxing, letting go, and experiencing an orgasm in front of their partner. On the flip side, it may be that women who find orgasms easy or satisfying interpret their enjoyable sex life as a sign of a strong, loving relationship. A study conducted by another research team, and also published in 2007, found somewhat similar results—specifically, that a person's sexual satisfaction was closely tied to the likelihood of orgasm, low conflict in a relationship, and high levels of intimacy.[10] The good news is that even if developing closeness and intimacy with a partner doesn't enhance your orgasm experience, it does promote general relationship satisfaction.

AN ORGASM-PRONE PERSONALITY?

A 2008 study of adult female twins living in the United Kingdom found that infrequent orgasms were linked to personality traits that included introversion, emotional instability, and not being open to new experiences.[11] These results, in conjunction with those of other studies that suggest a woman's frequency or ease of orgasm during intercourse is linked to genetics,[12] raise several important issues related to female orgasm. For example, to what extent does a woman's choice of partner influence her orgasmic experience? It may be that women who have genetic predispositions toward personality traits such as introversion choose partners with whom they are unlikely to develop emotionally close, supportive, or receptive relationships. Then again, it may be that women who are not open to new experiences (generally speaking) may also shy away from new sexual experiences, including those that may make it easier to experience more pleasurable or orgasmic sex. The more we learn about personality, partner selection, and orgasms, the more we can help direct women toward enjoyable (and orgasmic) solutions. Some women may find success learning to orgasm if they work on their relationship, whereas others may find it easier to orgasm if they focus on body self-exploration, self-pleasuring, or changes in sexual positions. Until we learn more, I hope that you will explore the whole range of strategies available to enhance your orgasmic ease and satisfaction.

MULTIPLE ORGASM

Although many women are interested in learning to have one orgasm, others are curious about the potential for having one orgasm after another: the so-called "multiple orgasm." Because so many women and men ask me about multiple orgasms, I'd be remiss if I didn't address the topic. The multiple orgasm is often described as the experience of having more than one orgasm during a sexual act, without losing one's arousal. Studies suggest that anywhere from 9 to 43 percent of women have had multiple orgasms (clearly, we need better research in this area!), but the vast majority of men are not capable of such a thing. Men have a refractory period, which is a period of time after they have ejaculated during which they cannot ejaculate again (often, they cannot get another firm erection during this time). Though we're not entirely sure what causes men's refractory period, we do know that it tends to lengthen with age, such that young men in their teens and twenties can often, as they say, go for two or more "rounds" of masturbation or sex in a row. While this isn't the same as multiple orgasm (since their arousal decreases in between each "round"), it is something that quite a few men and their partners enjoy. As men age, however, they may find that after having sex, it takes a full day before they are able to ejaculate again.

Many women, however, do seem capable of multiple orgasms throughout their lives. Like orgasms in general, multiple orgasms seem to get easier for women with time and experience. Often, women are curious about how multiple orgasms feel and whether each one feels progressively better. In fact,

Simultaneous Orgasm

The Hollywood version of sex often ends with both partners having powerful orgasms at exactly the same time. The reality, as you likely know, is much different. Though some couples strive to come at exactly the same time, most tend to take turns in a mutual sharing of pleasure—some because it is easier to orgasm one at a time and others because they enjoy focusing intently on each other and watching each other orgasm or experience pleasurable climactic sensations (but not necessarily orgasm). Do what feels enjoyable and natural to you, rather than what you see on-screen.

orgasms don't necessarily get stronger, more intense, or more pleasurable as a multiorgasmic experience progresses. Sometimes the first orgasm may be the most pleasurable or intense, and other times it may be a woman's second, third, or fourth orgasm in a row that she regards as most pleasurable.

We don't fully understand why some women experience multiple orgasms and others don't, though some women say that it is easier to do so during masturbation, vibrator use, or oral sex than it is during intercourse. After all, being able to have more than one orgasm requires a partner who is able and willing to continue having sex, and not all men are able to delay the timing of their ejaculation or get another erection after they ejaculate.

If you're interested in trying to have a second orgasm, try becoming highly—and I mean *very* highly—aroused before you even start having sex. Beginning from a point of intense pleasure and arousal can make both your first and second orgasm easier to achieve. Once you orgasm for the first time, there's no need to rush into a second attempt at orgasm right away unless your mind or body seem to be taking you in that direction. Instead, try relaxing for a moment, basking in the pleasure and euphoria of your orgasm, and then—when you (and your partner, if this is happening during partner sex) are ready—try moving your hips and stimulating your body in ways that feel good. This type of exploration may feel pleasurable (without leading to orgasm), or it may feel pleasurable in a way that suggests to you that another orgasm might indeed be possible.

Some women worry that if they wait to begin stimulation again, they will lose their arousal and the possibility of having an orgasm. In fact, though, it takes quite a while for physical arousal to subside—so if you'd like to enjoy your first orgasm for 3 seconds or a minute or two before starting stimulation again, feel free! This is *your* sexual experience, with time to explore.

THE OPTIONAL ORGASM

It is worth repeating that an orgasm is not a necessary or important part of feel-good sex for everyone. This is particularly true for women and men as they age and perhaps place an increased value on expressions of closeness and intimacy. Having an orgasm is an "optional" part of your overall sexual pleasure.

Taking such a perspective can, ironically, make it easier to experience an orgasm. When women are able to relax and enjoy sensual pleasures, they often find it easier to achieve an orgasm than when they are feeling tense or overly focused on having an orgasm. When we focus on the total experience—our feelings during the encounter, on the sensuality of being naked with someone we like, love, lust, and hopefully trust—we can experience intense levels of pleasure in line with little else in the world.

This may seem obvious on the surface, but stop and think about it for a moment. Remember the "cycles of dread"? Not only is it possible to get stuck in a cycle of dread when you have sex with a partner even though you don't feel like it, but it is also possible to dread sex when you begin viewing orgasms as something you "must" do or "should" experience. If you find that you are struggling with this issue and that your determination to have an orgasm is getting in the way of pleasurable, nourishing sex, please consider meeting with a sex therapist.

●

PRACTICING PLEASURE AND LEARNING TO ORGASM

There are many different activities and perspectives you can try that will help you ease your way toward experiencing pleasure and orgasms. Whether you want to shift your focus toward pleasure rather than orgasms, learn how to experience your first orgasm, or enhance your 500th orgasm, the suggestions below may be helpful to you. Additional tips and techniques are described in Chapter 8.

* **Experiment with your breathing.** During private or shared sex, try taking long, deep, slow breaths. Another time, try taking quick, shallow breaths, or hold your breath briefly (for just a few counts). How do these types of breathing affect your physical sensations? What about as your excitement builds, or as you approach orgasm? Does one type of breathing make it easier or more difficult to experience pleasure or to orgasm? How do they affect the intensity of your pleasure?

* **Change the pace of sex.** Some women find that although they enjoy one type of sex (such as rough or vigorous), they may orgasm more easily from a different sexual pace (such as slow or gentle). With your partner or alone, explore different paces of stimulation to see how they feel in terms of pleasure, excitement, intimacy, and ease of orgasm.

* **Be vocal!** Experiment with letting out moans of enjoyment. Try saying erotic words out loud, describing your fantasies to your partner, or letting him or her know what feels good, what you want more of, how to touch you, or what you're feeling. Research suggests that women who

✓ **FACT:** *Orgasm tends to become easier with age.*

The highest rates of orgasmic difficulty tend to be seen among those women who are relatively new to sex (those between the ages of 18 and 24). As women become more familiar with their bodies through self-pleasuring and partner play, as well as more practiced at their ability to communicate their desires and preferences for stimulation to a partner, they tend to find that they can orgasm with more ease and regularity.

✗ **MYTH:** *Orgasms always feel good.*

Though orgasms usually feel pleasurable, sometimes women experience pain in connection with orgasms. Menopausal women, for example, may notice pain in conjunction with the vaginal and uterine contractions that occur at the time of orgasm. (Hormonal treatment may help to address this problem.) Also, for reasons that remain unclear, some women may develop a sudden headache when they have an orgasm. If you experience pain in connection with orgasm, please consider checking in with your healthcare provider.

find it difficult to orgasm may be more likely to be in a relationship in which it is difficult for both partners to communicate about sexual activities that are likely to improve their orgasms. Talking openly about sex with one's partner may feel awkward at first, but it often grows easier with time.

�֍ **Self-pleasure.** If you're new to looking at (or sexually exploring) your genitals, by all means return to Chapter 2 as often as needed until you feel more comfortable touching your own body. As you explore, you may come across areas that respond strongly to touch, and as you grow more relaxed, that too can enhance your arousal and orgasm potential.

✱ **Just say no.** Although alcohol may help women and men to *feel* as though they are more sexually aroused, alcohol often impairs a person's physical arousal response. When that happens, it can feel considerably more difficult to reach orgasm. In the hours before sexual activity, choose nonalcoholic beverages so that you can make the most of your pleasure potential.

✱ **Hit the library!** One of my favorite books related to female orgasm is *Becoming Orgasmic: A Sexual and Personal Growth Program for Women* by Julia R. Heiman, PhD, of the Kinsey Institute, and Joseph LoPiccolo, PhD.[13] The tone is gentle and the information is enriching and of great importance, as the program detailed in the book has been shown to be highly effective in helping women learn to orgasm.

✱ **Get educated together.** Like women, many men have not received adequate education about women's bodies or sexual responses. Try not to blame your partner (or yourself) for his lack of knowledge, as it does not come naturally to anyone. Offer your support and work as a team to learn more together by reading books about female sexuality, partner sex, or relationship enhancement (see Resources on page 234).

✱ **Reposition yourself.** Think you've tried every possible sex position? Think again! Get out the *Kama Sutra* or the *Position of the Day Playbook* for radically different position ideas—or try slight variations on your old standbys. Hanging your head over the side of the bed during

●

missionary, for instance, can feel entirely different than propping it up on pillows. Changes to the angles of your hips or how close together (or apart) your legs are can affect sensation, too. The Coital Alignment Technique (CAT), in particular, has been shown to help women experience more pleasurable and orgasmic sex. (See Chapter 8 for details.)

✳ **Have a vivid fantasy life.** Men aren't the only visual creatures; women are, too. Though very few women experience orgasm from fantasies alone (meaning thoughts alone, with no touching involved), many more women find that fantasies can heighten their arousal, enhance their pleasure, and serve as an orgasm trigger. Give yourself permission to think erotic (and detailed) thoughts about your partner, neighbor, co-worker, or favorite celebrity—fantasy is a safe place where you can let go with abandon.

✳ **Keep an open mind.** The potential for orgasm can change in response to aging and life events. During pregnancy, a woman may find that her orgasms may become less frequent with each trimester, perhaps in part because pregnant women and their partners tend to spend less time in foreplay and intercourse, with less female-focused stimulation. Other women will find that their arousal and orgasmic abilities are enhanced during pregnancy, so try to keep an open mind about what sexual activity will be like for you during this time. Similarly, menopausal women tend to take longer for arousal-related changes (such as lubrication) to kick in, and they may experience less-intense orgasms than younger women. Yet, generally speaking, their sexual satisfaction (in spite of these orgasm changes) remains high—which goes to show that easy and strong orgasms are not always necessary for sexual satisfaction.

✳ **Play with toys.** Although masturbation exercises that involve one's hands are sufficiently enjoyable for many women as they explore pleasure and orgasms, some women find that using a sex toy such as a vibrator or dildo aids in their exploration. Vibrating sex toys can help some women learn to reach orgasm more quickly than they might without one. Others find that using a toy can help them feel sensation in their genitals more intensely; this may be particularly true for women who are in menopause, who have had a hysterectomy, or who have certain medical conditions associated with decreased bodily sensation. See Chapter 6 for more detailed information related to sex toys and sexual enhancement.

FEMALE EJACULATION

Although the term "female ejaculation" is commonly used to refer to fluids that are expelled (or seemingly "squirt") from a woman's urethra during sexual arousal or orgasm, both the term and the act that it describes remain controversial. There has only been a little bit of research in this area, and it hasn't illuminated this phenomenon as much as many of us wish. What we do know is that women describe a range of feelings of wetness during sexual activity. Some feel mild vaginal wetness, while others report larger amounts of fluids that are emitted from the urethra or vagina, either gradually throughout sex or suddenly all at once. For many of these women, the fluids are expelled at the point of orgasm; others notice them after several minutes of G-spot stimulation or when they are feeling very aroused (but not in association with orgasm). As far as what exactly the fluid is, the results are mixed: In four studies, chemical tests showed that these sexual fluids expelled by women were distinctly different from urine. Two other studies failed to find such differences, and it is certainly possible that some women—such as those who experience stress urinary incontinence—may leak urine during sexual activity.

In many cases, a woman can investigate this herself. If you're concerned that you leak urine during sexual excitement or arousal, try placing a white sheet or towel underneath you during masturbation and check the color or smell of the fluids in question to see if they are similar to urine. If not, and if you have no other reason to believe that you're leaking urine (if you don't leak urine in response to laughing or sneezing, or at other times), then perhaps you can chalk up your response to being similar to many other women who experience female ejaculation—or whatever you feel like calling it. Many couples find it sexy or arousing when a woman becomes very wet during sex, and your partner may take your wetness as a welcome sign that you're feeling very turned-on by your shared sexual experience. If, however, the wetness bothers either of you, consider laying a towel down on the bed or keeping one nearby for easy cleanup. If the color or odor are similar to urine or if you are concerned that you may indeed be leaking urine during sex, check in with your healthcare provider; he or she may be able to offer treatment.

HOMEWORK
What Makes Sex Good?

Think about for a moment—or list in the space below—your favorite things about being sexual with another person. Try to think of at least four, if possible.

FAVORITE THINGS

1. _____

2. _____

3. _____

4. _____

Usually when I ask women and men to try this exercise, few of the responses have anything to do with orgasm. Rather, the vast majority of people's favorite parts of sex have to do with kissing, touching, feeling warm, cuddling, laughing together, and seeing a side of a person that no one else ever gets to see. As you now know from reading this chapter, these responses reflect what research typically finds—that although orgasm is enjoyed by many women and men, the broader sexual experience and the intimacy between the two people sharing it are more closely linked with satisfaction and pleasure than orgasm is.

On a related note, several years ago, researchers in the Netherlands interviewed 8- and 9-year-old children (both boys and girls) about what it felt like for them to "fall in love" with or develop crushes on other children.[14] The children tended to describe their feelings of liking and love in positive terms, including that it felt "nice" and "fun." However, my two favorite descriptions were from children who described being in love as feeling like "a tickling sensation" and something that "makes you feel proud." To me, these findings reflect our lifelong propensity for valuing the emotional aspects of intimacy at least as much, if not more than, the physical sensations that, as adults, we experience as part of sex.

Sex Toys

*Your Guide to the Basics
and the Best*

Over the past decade, sex toys have become increasingly mainstream and available to both women and men in the United States and around the world. Though not everyone prefers the term "sex toy," I do, because it makes me think about the fun, playful, pleasurable aspects of sex that sometimes fall by the wayside when pleasurable sex becomes "duty" sex. Other terms you may hear for sex toys include "sexual aids," "sexual enhancement products," "bedroom toys," or "bedroom accessories." No term is more technically correct or accurate than the others—use the words that make you feel comfortable.

In this chapter, I want to provide you with information about sex toys and the women and men who use them, including how these products can be used to address issues related to arousal, desire, and orgasm. I'll also share important safety and hygiene guidelines that you should consider before you use or purchase any product. But before we go any further, let's begin with our quiz.

POP QUIZ

1. Why were electric vibrators first invented?

    a. To give women orgasms when their partners could not

    b. To pleasure women who did not have partners

    c. To provide "medical" treatment for women

    d. To try to locate the elusive G-spot

2. What percentage of American women, ages 18 to 60, have *ever* used a vibrator during masturbation or sex with a partner?

    a. 20%

    b. 33%

    c. 40%

    d. 53%

3. Which of the following is one of the easiest sex toy materials to keep clean?

    a. Silicone

    b. "Jelly" (PVC)

    c. Leather

    d. Latex

4. Which of the following is an advantage of "glass" dildos?

    a. They can be cleaned in the dishwasher.

    b. They can be warmed or cooled by running them under water.

⚬

c. They can be used to provide more "firm" stimulation than softer sex toys.

d. They are less porous than other materials and thus easier to keep clean.

e. All of the above.

Answers: 1) c; 2) d; 3) a; 4) e

When I talk about sex toys, I'm referring to products such as vibrators, dildos, c-rings (also called cock rings), clitoral pumps, anal toys, and men's masturbation sleeves. Some of these toys are intended to be used by women (privately or with a partner); others are meant to be used by men or couples. Though sex toys may seem like an invention of modern times, they have actually been around for many generations and were used by people of many cultures including Egyptians, Greeks, Chinese, Japanese, and Europeans. At the Kinsey Institute, we have erotic art images in our collection originating from 19th-century Japan, China, and France (as well as from more contemporary times) including those that depict women, men, couples, singles, and groups using objects as dildos. Similar art and artifacts can be found in museums and galleries around the world, as well as on the Internet.

Today numerous products are sold as sex toys through venues such as women's in-home sex toy parties (similar to Tupperware or Mary Kay parties, except in-home sex toy parties sell vibrators and other sex toys, not resealable containers or makeup), boutiques, the Internet (including mainstream sites like Amazon.com), adult bookstores, drug stores, and retail chains. During the past decade, the sex toy industry has become so mainstream that you can now buy

●

lubricants and vibrating toys in some drug stores and learn about the latest, greatest vibrator from Oprah Winfrey's *O, The Oprah Magazine.*

For years, I've collaborated with sex toy manufacturers, distributors, engineers, and designers on research, consulting, and education projects. I've even helped to design sex toys for various companies. I've assisted with designing these products because I value the quality and safety of the products that make their way onto the shelves of stores and into the hands (and other parts!) of consumers like you and me. For too many years, low-quality products made up the bulk of toys. Now, things are changing.

Whether you're new to sex toys or have already experimented with them, I think you'll learn a few things and maybe even become inspired to use them in new, more pleasurable ways. By the end of this chapter, I hope that you will feel comfortable:

✱ Looking at and reading about sex toys on the Internet, in a woman-friendly sex toy shop, at an in-home sex toy party, or in a local store

✱ Choosing a sex toy that feels right to you (that is, if you're interested in trying a toy; not everyone is, and that is absolutely okay) and using it in pleasurable ways

✱ Talking to your partner (if you have one) about sex toys and whether toys are something you are interested in using as a couple, and possibly using one together

✱ Sharing your own and listening to your friends' experiences, thoughts, and opinions related to sex toys. Even if you and your friends choose not to share intimate information, you might laugh about the episode of

Sex and the City where Charlotte bought a Rabbit vibrator. Or you can tell your friends what you've learned about sex toys by reading this book, and ask what they think.

Of course, using a vibrator or other sex toy is a personal decision and is not for everyone. Just as some women like to grind their own coffee rather than use an electric coffee maker, some women prefer to touch or rub their own bodies with their hands (or against a partner's body) rather than use an electric or battery-powered vibrator. Put another way, women who walk to work can arrive on time just as easily as women who use modern technology (such as cars or the subway) do—it's just that one woman may get there a little faster than the other.

Safety Tips for Sharing Sex Toys

✱ Don't do it. I mean, why, people? There are many affordable toys out there—spring for two!

✱ If you decide that you *must* share, clean the toy before and after each person's use, put a new condom on the toy before it touches your body, and then remove it and put on another new condom before it touches your partner's body.

✱ You did both get tested for sexually transmissible diseases (STDs) before deciding to share toys, right?

✱ Guys: If you're trying to impress a new lady friend, please note that keeping a vibrator in your nightstand does not spell "prepared" or "thoughtful"—it screams, "Gross, where else has that been?" Instead, if you're aiming to share the vibration love, consider buying single-use vibrating condom rings (because you *are* using condoms with new or uncommitted partners, right?). Affordable and safe!

Neither is better or worse; they are simply different ways of doing the same thing.

As such, you have numerous options when it comes to self-pleasuring or partner play. You can use a vibrator, dildo, or your hand to stimulate your genitals, or you can rub against a bed or pillow as a means of self-stimulation. You might aim the water from the bathtub faucet toward your genitals, touch your breasts, or sensuously graze your inner thighs with your fingers. Then again, you might not self-pleasure your body in any sexual way whatsoever. Your sexual play might be entirely with a partner, and not with yourself. Although masturbation is common among both single and coupled women, it is certainly not a "must" and you should do only what feels good for you.

Some women wonder whether it is common to masturbate. Studies consistently confirm that, regardless of age, religion, or relationship status, it is very common. Not only have most women masturbated at some point in their lives, but many—nearly half of women, according to some research—have masturbated as recently as the previous month. Like men, women masturbate for a variety of reasons, the most popular of which are of the "feel-good" variety—namely, to have an orgasm and to experience sexual pleasure. Relieving sexual tension and relaxing are other commonly offered reasons.

WHO USES SEX TOYS—AND WHY?

Okay, you might be thinking, so women masturbate. But that doesn't mean that they all use vibrators or other sex toys while self-pleasuring—does it? It's true that some women self-pleasure with water dripping from their bathtub faucet, by

FACT: *The electric vibrator was invented as a medical treatment for women's hysteria.*

True story! According to historian Rachel Maines,[1] hysteria—a diagnosis given exclusively to women for any number of symptoms including exhaustion, nervousness, and abdominal heaviness (but recognized by some as sexual deprivation)—was often treated with "pelvic massage," which was actually vaginal massage, administered by doctors or midwives. The diagnosis of hysteria—and its treatments—seem to have been relatively common throughout history and certainly occurred in the United States in the 1800s and early 1900s. Treatment often left the "patient" feeling calmer and relaxed (satisfied)—and kept them coming back, since these treatments weren't necessarily regarded as sexual. After all, "sex" meant intercourse, not genital touching. Though treatment for this chronic condition was profitable for healthcare providers of the time, it was also time-consuming. The invention of the electromechanical vibrator in the late 1800s, however, allowed first for more rapid office treatments and, later on, for women to "treat" themselves at home. Though women have been using vibrators for more than a century now, only recently have they become commonplace, openly discussed, and even fashionable.

MYTH: *Vibrators are addictive.*

While I am often asked about whether you can become "addicted" to vibrators, I am pretty much never asked whether you can become addicted to oral sex, vaginal or anal intercourse—or massaging shower-heads, for that matter. Why are people so nervous about becoming dependent on vibrators? They are simply sexual enhancement aids that many women find pleasurable to use, and therefore may do so regularly. But they're certainly not "addictive." Coffee and soda are more habit-forming than vibrators!

rubbing against a bed, while reading erotic stories, or (unintentionally) through a pleasantly surprising "orgasmic dream" in the middle of the night. However, many women do use sex toys and, as people tend to be curious about what their friends, family members, and neighbors are up to behind closed doors, we asked. In 2008, our research team at the Center for Sexual Health Promotion at Indiana University, Bloomington, surveyed more than 2,000 women and more than 1,000 men between the ages of 18 and 60. We asked the participants about their sexual experiences and their use of sexual enhancement products. We found that nearly half (47 percent) of women had used a vibrator during masturbation and, when we included those who had ever used a vibrator during sex with a partner, the figure jumped to 53 percent.[2] In case you're curious about the men, though they more often had used a vibrator with a partner than during masturbation, nearly half of them had used a vibrator alone or with a partner.

No wonder vibrators have wound up on the pages of everything from women's magazines like *Cosmopolitan* to the *New York Times*—we women (and our partners) can't seem to get enough of them. At the very least, we're curious.

Why did people start using vibrators in the first place? Were they lonely, desperate, or otherwise out of luck in their sex lives? Far from it! If anything, women and men tend to say that they started using vibrators for fun, out of curiosity, to make it easier for themselves (or their partner) to have an orgasm, or to otherwise spice up their sex lives. In other words, these are people who, like you and me, are interested in pleasure, enjoyment, and satisfaction.

While some people have stereotypical ideas about what

•

vibrator users are like, our research suggests that women and men who use vibrators, whether alone or with a partner, are similar to those who don't: They are typically healthy, well-balanced individuals from all walks of life. They may be diverse in terms of age, race, ethnicity, and sexual orientation, and they may (or may not) be in a relationship or married. It doesn't matter whether they identify as moderate, liberal, or conservative; whether they went to college, earned a graduate degree, or went to work (or started a family) straight out of high school: Vibrator use is common.

WAIT, THERE'S MORE!

Although vibrators are enjoyed by many women and men worldwide, they are far from the only type of sexual enhancement product used by individuals or couples. Lubricant is commonly used to enhance sex (about 70 percent of Americans have used a lubricant during sex), and we now have more lubricant choices than ever, including those that are warming, hypoallergenic, flavored, or organic. Then there are condoms that are ribbed, studded, coated with warming lubricant, or that have a baggy end to enhance sensation—all of which are purchased with the goal of making sex feel more fun, erotic, or rich with sensation. Like lubricants, many condoms are considered sexual enhancement products. (And if you ask me, even the most basic condoms can be considered sexual enhancement products because they can improve sex by making it safer and thus more relaxing for couples.) You can learn more about lubricants in this chapter, as well as in Chapters 4 and 8.

TOUR OF TOYS

Given that there are hundreds, if not thousands, of toy types, I won't be able to cover them all in this chapter. However, for the toy-curious reader, the following information will arm you with plenty of knowledge of both the basic and the newer, more cutting-edge toys.

External-Use Toys

Although many people describe these toys as "clitoral toys," not everyone uses them directly on the glans clitoris (the part one can see from the outside). Some people use these toys to stimulate the breasts or nipples, perianal area, or a man's penis or scrotum. Also, they may be used for masturbation, couples play, or intercourse, but what separates them from other toys is that they are not intended or recommended for internal (meaning vaginal or anal) use; they are generally seen as "external use only" toys.

Bullets: Usually made from hard plastic and coated with a silver sheen—and therefore called "silver bullets"—vibrating bullets (see below) often have multiple speeds, which is useful for beginners and experienced sex toy users alike. Women new

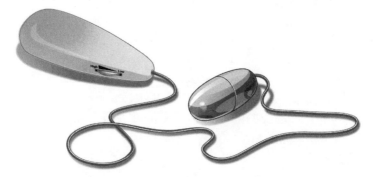

Silver bullet vibrator

to toys may be unsure which level of intensity they'll prefer, and experienced toy users may already know that they enjoy different intensities at different points during the sexual experience (such as low intensity to encourage desire or build arousal, followed by a higher intensity to encourage climax or orgasm). Bullets are nearly always powered by standard AA or AAA batteries, are widely available, and—as a bonus—are typically quite affordable.

Hitachi Magic Wand: This toy was made famous by Betty Dodson, a long-time advocate of women's sexual pleasure and author of *Sex for One: The Joy of Selfloving*,[3] who has taught hands-on masturbation workshops to women. The Wand (see below) is often sold as a body massager, but many women and men have found more intimate uses for this vibrating toy. Various attachments are available, which adds to the diverse ways in which one can use this electric-powered (wall plug-in) toy for masturbation.

Finger vibrators: Given the number of women who crave a vibrator that is small enough to fit in between two bodies

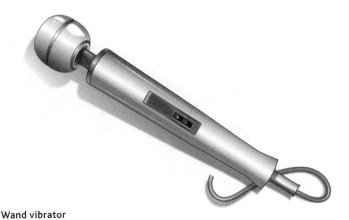

Wand vibrator

during intercourse—and stimulate the clitoris without being obtrusive—it is no wonder that women and men are curious about finger vibrators. Such toys fit over your finger, almost as an extension of the finger, for targeted stimulation of your chosen body part.

Clitoral pumps: These devices may be sold as either vibrating or nonvibrating toys. One version, the NuGyn Eros Therapy device, has been approved by the U.S. Food and Drug Administration (FDA) for the treatment of female sexual dysfunction (namely for problems related to difficulty with arousal and orgasm) and is available by prescription. Note how clinical-sounding the name is—it's a "device," not a "toy," and it's for "therapy," not "pleasure." Okay, we get it. Product name aside, the Eros has been shown to aid in women's sexual arousal, lubrication, satisfaction, and genital sensation. Novelty companies sell similar products, but the imitations have not been tested so it's unclear to what extent they help women with similar concerns or whether they are "just" for fun and pleasure. (We like pleasure!)

Laya: Considering the number of women who work on computers all day and may suffer from tendinitis or carpal tunnel syndrome, it was about time that someone made a vibrating toy with ergonomics and wrist issues in mind. Enter the Laya, a toy that is gently curved so that women can lie on it rather than hold it against their genitals.

SaSi: A relatively new product, the SaSi is intended for stimulating the clitoris and/or vaginal opening (not way inside, just the immediate vaginal entrance). What's cutting-edge about the SaSi, however, is that some women swear it feels similar to cunnilingus. Also you can actually "teach" the vibrating toy what you like by rotating through various speed

●

and directional patterns and then pressing the "Don't Stop" button to indicate that you want a particular pattern to be used again and again in the future. Yes, that's right: a sex toy that you can train!

Vibrating Vaginal Toys

Toys intended to stimulate the vagina generally fall into one of four subcategories: slimline or phallic vibrators, eggs, G-spot vibrators, and dual (or triple) action vibrators.

Slimline or phallic vibrators: These vibrating toys may be made to look like a penis (phallic) or they may be long, smooth, and cylindrical (the classic slimline types) (see below).

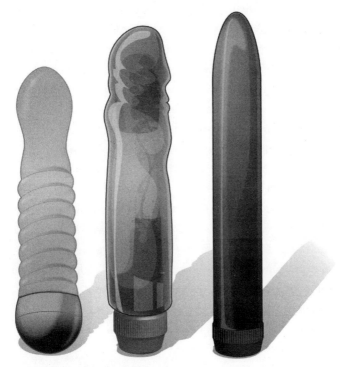

Slimline and phallic vibrators

These are what many women and men often imagine when they think of traditional vibrators.

Eggs: Vibrating eggs are vibrators that are inserted vaginally, but they are curiously shaped like chicken eggs and thus can enhance a woman's feeling of vaginal fullness. Some varieties are remote-controlled and can be turned on by a woman's partner from a range of 50 feet! What, you might wonder, would couples do with such a toy? As a means of sexual play and arousal, a woman can insert the vibrating egg, give her partner the remote, and then he can turn the egg on and off from as close as across a restaurant dinner table or as far as the next room (thus stimulating a woman's vagina from a distance). It can be an exciting private secret for a couple to share as foreplay or sex play. If you've never been teased by a little unexpected vibration over wine and dessert, you may be surprised to find how sexy and fun it can be. (No worries about it slipping out unexpectedly, either; it's inserted several inches back, like a tampon, and stays securely in place.)

G-spot vibrators: According to research conducted by our team at the Center for Sexual Health Promotion, women have many questions about G-spot vibrators, which reflects women's overall curiosity about the G-spot (see Chapters 2 and 8). The main difference between G-spot toys and slimline/phallic toys is that G-spot vibrators, as well as nonvibrating G-spot dildos, are curved in a way that makes it easier to target stimulation toward the front wall of the vagina for G-spot stimulation (see opposite page). That said, if you find that G-spot stimulation doesn't do much for you, you can always use your toy to stimulate other parts of your vagina, vulva (including the clitoris), breasts, or your partner's body.

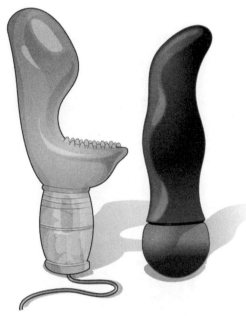

G-spot vibrators

Dual- (or triple-) action toys: These are multipurpose—they're usually built to stimulate a woman's glans clitoris and her vagina simultaneously. That said, some stimulate the vagina and anus, while others (the triple-action types) can simultaneously stimulate the clitoris, vagina, and anus. Talk about multitasking! More advanced models may have switches that allow users to keep one part vibrating (for example, the clitoral stimulator) while another part (such as the vaginal stimulator) stays quietly stationary (without vibrating). Versions of the aforementioned Rabbit vibrator (made famous on the television show *Sex and the City*) fall into this category. Some dual-action toys may have rotating balls inside the shaft, and if you look closely, you'll notice that the balls tend to be focused only in the toy's first few

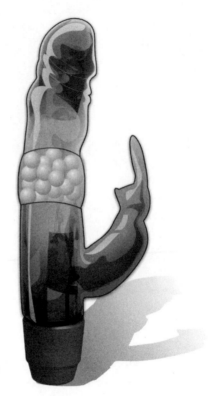

Dual action vibrator

inches (see above); that's because the lower part of the vagina appears to be more sensitive than the upper portion is. (This is why when a tampon is positioned toward the back of the vagina, a woman can usually not feel it inside of her.) Some newer models even have "thrusting" movements that make the top part of the vaginal vibrator grow in length.

Nonvibrating Vaginal Toys

Dildos: Some women, including those who would like to learn to orgasm from vaginal intercourse or whose genitals are uncomfortably sensitive to vibration, prefer to use dildos (see opposite page).

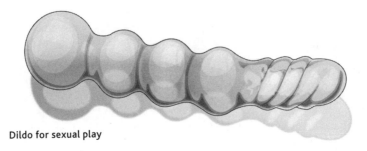

Dildo for sexual play

Unlike vibrators, dildos are nearly always waterproof, since they don't have battery compartments or motors. Dildos may be made from a range of materials such as rubber, plastic, steel, or soft glass (which is actually a hard, thick glass that's more like Pyrex, so no worries about it breaking inside you!) or even beautifully crafted hardwood. (And yes, I totally get the irony of having a hardwood dildo.)

Couples Toys

Though most sex toys can be used by couples in creative, arousing ways, some toys are specifically designed with vaginal intercourse in mind.

Partner rings: Available through many in-home parties and sex boutiques, partner rings typically feature flexible c-rings that fit snugly around a man's penis and scrotum (thus providing firm stimulation) while anchoring a small vibrating silver bullet at the base of the penis that, during vaginal intercourse, is positioned brilliantly to stimulate a woman's glans clitoris. It's important to note that healthcare providers generally recommend that men wear c-rings for no longer than 20 minutes, so as to allow blood to flow in and out of the penis without constriction. Also, men should remove rings if they feel uncomfortable, feel pain, or experience bruising of the penis or scrotum. While these risks are very rare, they are important to be aware of, especially for men who have thicker penises.

Vibrating condom rings: Available online as well as through some drug stores and retail chains, these are essentially smaller, tamer, disposable versions of partner rings. Vibrating condom rings typically feature one ring instead of two and fit around the base of a man's penis. If a man is wearing a condom, then the ring slips over the condom and helps to hold it securely on the base of his penis. It simultaneously stimulates a woman's clitoris during intercourse thanks to a small vibrating piece anchored at the base of the penis. Be aware, though, that many vibrating rings only last for 15 to 20 minutes, and many women may require additional stimulation in order to orgasm. As a reminder, these rings should be worn for no more than 20 minutes.

We-Vibe: In 2008, the We-Vibe arrived on the scene (see below). Made of medical-grade silicone, it's easy to clean and can be worn by a woman during vaginal intercourse. Its U shape

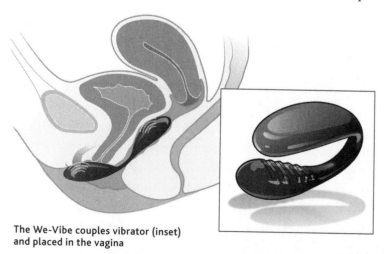

The We-Vibe couples vibrator (inset)
and placed in the vagina

allows one branch to stimulate a woman's vagina (and, during intercourse, her partner's penis) while the other branch stimulates her clitoral area and mons pubis. Though a couple may need to adjust their lovemaking a bit to use the toy, a little creativity never hurt anyone. Some couples find that rear entry is more comfortable with the We-Vibe than missionary is, as the man's body can uncomfortably press the toy against a woman's pubic bone in missionary. See Chapter 8 for tips on how to pleasurably use the We-Vibe with a partner.

Boy Toys Used for Partner Play

Sleeves: Also known as "penis sleeves" or "masturbation sleeves," these are toys that men may use during solo masturbation in various positions (standing, sitting, or lying down). Many sleeves depict molded shapes of a woman's lips, vulva, or butt to inspire men's fantasies. Some women find it pleasurable to masturbate their partner with a sleeve or to incorporate one into intercourse, particularly if their partner is well endowed or they're simply looking to spice things up. (See Chapter 8 for a how-to.)

Penis extenders: These are toys that a man slips over his penis and uses during intercourse to add length or girth (see page 142). Sheaths tend to be thinner versions of extenders and may allow more sensation for the man while still adding girth for female pleasure. Ticklers (nonvibrating toys that may also be called "enhancers") tend to be wider than vibrating condom rings and fit over a man's penis as a cross between a ring and a sheath. Their intent is to add girth to a man's penis for added stimulation of his female partner *without* entirely covering a man's penis (which sheaths and extenders often do). Some ticklers feature ridges or "nubbies" (raised circles or prickly

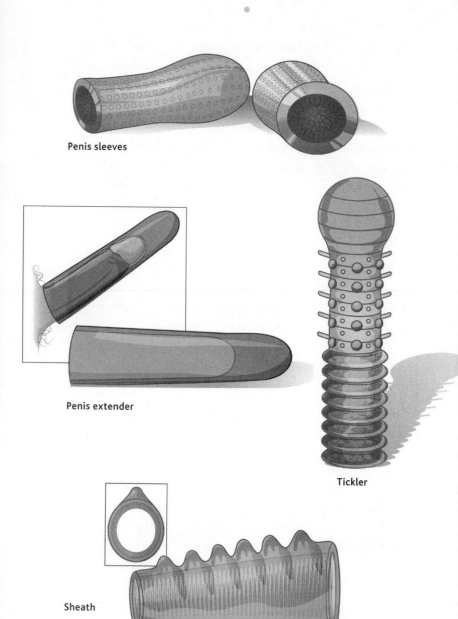

Penis sleeves

Penis extender

Tickler

Sheath

bits of material) to stimulate either partner during intercourse. Each of these toys is most comfortably used with a fair amount of lubricant (a nickel- or dime-size amount).

C-rings: When discussing partner rings and vibrating condom rings above, I alluded to c-rings (also called cock rings or erection rings). These may be structured as double or single rings. Single rings stretch to fit over the base of the penis; double rings fit over the base of the penis and also a man's scrotum. Either one may offer firm but gentle stimulation to a man's body. Although these toys are often used to help men maintain an erection, there is very little scientific data to support that they are actually capable of doing so; as such, they should be regarded as more of a novelty item than an erectile aid. Again, the 20-minute time limit applies.

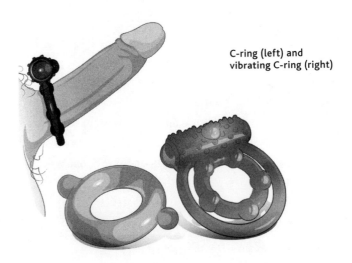

C-ring (left) and
vibrating C-ring (right)

WHAT TOYS ARE MADE OF: THE BASICS

Just as it is important to know that silk clothes, while attractive, can easily stain and may be expensive to clean, and cotton, while comfy, can shrink in the wash, understanding some basic info about sex toy materials can help you purchase toys that will fit in with your lifestyle and keep you safe from health hazards. That said, there are numerous materials used in toys and this is just a sampling of the more commonly used materials—others may be made of metal, vinyl, acrylic, Lucite, leather, wood, or combinations of materials. If it is unclear what the toy you're shopping for is made of, please ask or e-mail a customer service representative so that you know what you're putting on or inside your body and how best to clean it. Sex toys are generally constructed of one of the following materials.

* **Silicone:** Toys made of medical-grade silicone are generally regarded as soft, smooth, easy to clean, nontoxic, and hypoallergenic. (People rarely have allergic reactions to silicone products.) But let the buyer beware: "Silicone-based" toys may not always have much silicone in them—they may also contain PVC, natural rubber, latex, or other chemicals. Look for toys made of medical-grade silicone or made by manufacturers that provide information about any other materials used in the toy's construction.

* **Rubber:** Many sex toys are made of latex rubber, which is inexpensive, thus making these products affordable. On the downside, people with latex allergies should steer clear of rubber toys (or any toy whose chemical makeup they are uncertain about).

✱ **Jelly:** Though often among the most affordable toys, those described as "jelly" are often made with polyvinyl chloride (PVC), a plastic that can leach potentially toxic chemicals into the body. The use of PVC in vaginal sex toys is controversial for this reason. In tests conducted by the Danish Environmental Protection Agency, toys described as "jelly" often contained phthalates, which are chemicals that may be toxic or potentially harmful (perhaps especially for women who are pregnant or breastfeeding). I suggest that you consider using other toys or use a barrier method by slipping a condom over a "jelly" toy. Using a water-based lubricant with these toys also may pose less of a risk than using oil-based lubricants, according to preliminary research. Another con to jelly toys? They sometimes give off a plasticlike odor—not sexy.

✱ **Plastic:** *The Graduate* gave us more than just Mrs. Robinson—it also highlighted the "great future in plastics!" Though nowhere near lifelike in terms of their

Storing Your Toys

Just because you feel comfortable with your sex life doesn't mean that toys should be left out in the open. If a sex toy has small parts or attachments and you have children, please store the toy in a childproof cupboard or out of reach. Some companies sell pillows or stylish cases in which you can store your toy out of sight from visiting neighbors or the in-laws. To keep your vibrators running longer, remove the batteries after each use. Finally, jelly (PVC) toys may melt in hot temperatures or even seep into each other if they are stored close together; instead, store them separately in individual plastic or fabric bags.

●

feel, hard plastic toys are often affordable and easy to clean. Common types of plastic toys include slimline vibrators and silver bullets. An added bonus to plastic toys is that they transmit vibration intensely, albeit a bit loudly.

* **CyberSkin:** Quite soft and (some say) closer to the feeling of human skin, preliminary research suggests that toys made of CyberSkin pose no unusual risks in terms of toxicity. The material can feel warm and lifelike with use but, on the downside, can be a little pricey.

* **Glass:** Think Pyrex, rather than windowpanes. These popular glass toys (sold as dildos, and rarely as vibrators) are smooth, solid masses that you can cool down or warm up by running them under cool or warm water. They are easily cleaned and can provide firmer vaginal stimulation than toys made of softer materials.

CLEANING YOUR SEX TOY

Since you can't send sex toys to the dry cleaner, you must clean them yourself. Because cleaning methods vary based on the toy, always ask the person who sells you a toy for detailed information about how it should be cleaned. Most toys can be cleaned with warm water and soap, but vibrators cannot safely be held under water unless they are waterproof. (Always keep water and soap away from batteries, battery compartments, and electrical components such as wiring.) If a toy is not waterproof, you can often take a damp cloth or cotton ball soaked in soap and water (or rubbing alcohol) and clean the toy by hand. Commercially sold sex toy cleaner can be sprayed on most toys, too.

Glass dildos may be cleaned in the dishwasher or sink.

Men's masturbation sleeves, as they don't have motors, can also be cleaned with water. Medical-grade silicone dildos (but not vibrators) can even be boiled in a pot of water on the stove—but I don't recommend it, particularly as some toys that are described as "silicone" contain other materials that may melt or degrade in hot water.

Cleaning your sex toy is important. If you don't clean toys properly after each use, they can harbor bacteria and increase your chances of a urinary tract infection (UTI), bacterial imbalance in the vagina, or genital irritation. If you have special concerns or needs related to hygiene (like if you have a compromised immune system due to illness or medical treatments), you may want to take an extra precaution and put a condom over your toy prior to use, and check in with your healthcare provider for cleaning recommendations.

CHOOSING A LUBRICANT FOR TOY PLAY

Many women find that adding a lubricant makes toy play more comfortable, pleasurable, and satisfying. There are a variety of

Side Effects?

Like vaginal and anal intercourse, sex toys present a small risk of "side effects" such as genital irritation, itching, inflammation, or even small cuts or tears (particularly if one's genital skin is thin or vulnerable due to preexisting hormonal or skin conditions). If you experience uncomfortable or worrisome genital symptoms due to using sex toys, or due to intercourse, masturbation, or other sex play, please check in with your healthcare provider. Sex injuries occasionally occur and some require medical care.

•

Undercover Lovers

Not all toys scream "sex!" Some vibrators masquerade as rubber ducky bath toys, hairbrushes, MP3 players, and tubes of lipstick. (See "Woman-Friendly Online Sex Toy Shops and Boutiques" on page 240 for more info.)

options available, and it can be confusing to know which one is right for you. Here's a breakdown of the benefits and drawbacks of each of the basic formulas.

* **Water-based lubricants** can be used with the vast majority of toys but are best for sex that occurs "on land"—as in not in the shower or bath, where it can easily wash away, leaving you lube-free and potentially feeling dry.

* **Silicone-based lubricants** may be more expensive than other varieties, but they provide long-lasting lubrication (perfect for marathon sex sessions) and won't wash off easily, so they're ideal for sex or toy play in the bath or shower. That said, silicone lube may damage silicone toys, so if your toy is silicone, consider pairing it with a water-based lube or putting a condom over the toy and then adding silicone lubricant to the condom.

* **Oil-based lubricants** are rarely recommended for sex or toy play. That's because they can cause latex condoms to break or tear and may increase your risk of exposure to toxic chemicals in some sex toy materials. However, an oil-based lubricant may be a good option for you during intercourse with a monogamous partner with whom you don't use condoms.

If you have questions about personal health issues and lubricants, please check in with your healthcare provider. Also, see Chapter 8 for more information about lubricants, including special considerations for women's health issues.

BOY MEETS TOY

Although women in same-sex relationships are often toy-friendly, many women in heterosexual relationships wonder if their male partner will be open to their desire to use a vibrator or other sex toy. In my experience, I've found that the vast majority of men feel comfortable with—or turned on by—the prospect of a partner using a sex toy or participating in sex toy play. That said, using sex toys doesn't come naturally to most people, and some men may be intimidated at first. When a woman is interested in bringing her sex toy and her partner closer, I generally suggest the following tips.

Splish, Splash!

If you're curious about trying out your favorite sex toy in a bathtub, shower, or hot tub, make sure that it's safe to use underwater. Most nonvibrating dildos can be used under water. Waterproof vibrators have an extra seal indicating that they are safe to get wet (which makes them a particularly good choice for women who experience female ejaculation during excitement or orgasm and who don't want to worry about keeping their toys dry during the throes of passion). Because warm water can dry out the vagina, silicone lubricants are often recommended for underwater sexploration; they'll make penetration more comfortable and pleasurable.

1. **Choose a comfortable time to talk.** Find a time when you're not having—or about to have—sex, and talk to your partner about sex toys. Ask how he feels about using them and whether he'd be open to using one with you. Share ideas about what would feel comfortable and pleasurable about using toys together, as well as any concerns or boundaries that you might have. If you need an opening, start by saying that you read about toys in a book (like this one!) or magazine and it made you curious about how he'd feel using one together.

2. **Focus on the pluses.** As with anything new, focus on the bright side and what it will bring to your sex life. Has he expressed a desire to learn how to make it easier for you to orgasm? Offer to show him how you use your sex toy. Perhaps he's curious about what it will do for him, too. You might mention that some men can feel the vibration during intercourse when a vibrator is held to a woman's clitoris, and that vibration can sometimes enhance a man's erection and orgasm, too.

3. **Show him examples.** If he's feeling iffy about sex toys, you might sit together and browse the sex toys that are for sale on couples-friendly Web sites (see the Resources on page 234).

Famous Fans of Sex Toys

Sex toys are no longer a secret—thanks in part to sex-positive celebrities such as Eva Longoria, Kim Cattrall, Missy Elliot, Jenny McCarthy, and Teri Hatcher, who have talked, written, or sang about vibrators. Other high-profile women, such as Halle Berry and Kate Middleton, have been spotted at sex toy shops or parties, or otherwise been rumored to have made a vibrating purchase. (Whether or not it's true is anybody's guess.)

●

Sex Ed

Stay up-to-date on the newest, most innovative (and safest) sex toys by checking out my Web site, www.MySexProfessor.com. Browse the archives to read my reviews and ratings of women's, men's, and couples' toys.

This can be a nonthreatening way to get familiar with toys and share thoughts and ideas about which toys are within your comfort zone as a couple. You might also volunteer to show him the toy that you use—sometimes fear lies in the unknown, and seeing an actual toy may help to demystify any concerns.

4. **Read a book together!** Your partner may find this chapter a particularly interesting read, given the expanded range of sex toys—after all, many men love gadgets, and some of these toys are interesting if for no other reason than that they are technological innovations! *The Good Vibrations Guide to Sex* by Cathy Winks and Anne Semans[4] is another book that illustrates how couples can incorporate sex toys into their shared sex life.

HOMEWORK
A Babe in Toyland

Choose one (or both) of these two toy activities to enhance your sex toy comfort level and knowledge.

1. If you're new to toys, here's your chance to embark on a Sex Toy Scavenger Hunt to learn more about them. Go online and browse through sites that sell sex toys and see if you can find a Web site from which you would feel comfortable learning about or even buying a sex toy. What do you like or dislike about the way that some Web sites look compared to others? Which sites provide detailed information about sex toys (like how to clean them or use them with a partner)? Are there other "accessories," such as condoms, lubricants, or sex toy cleaners that the sites sell, too, and that might enhance your sexual experience? To discover what's in your own backyard, carry your scavenger hunt to a local adult bookstore or woman-oriented sex toy boutique, or attend an in-home sex toy party. Ask yourself similar questions about how you feel about the look and feel of the shop or party, and the chance to touch or turn on sex toys and other enhancement products. If you were to buy a sex toy, where would you feel most comfortable? And how would you feel shopping for a toy with a friend or partner?

2. If you're a seasoned sex toy veteran, consider using this opportunity for sex toy exploration. Try using your favorite toy in new and interesting ways. Even if you think you've done everything with it, certainly there is something new you can try. If you generally use your toy alone, consider using it with a partner (or letting your partner use it on you in the dark or while blindfolded). Do you normally press your toy against your bare genitals? Try using it while you're fully clothed or in your underwear. Used to dry land? Take a waterproof toy into the bath. If you're all about high intensity, try a lower intensity to allow your excitement to build gradually over time. There are numerous ways to use toys alone or with a partner, and many new and inventive toys are on the market, so there's no excuse not to try something new and learn what it might add to your pleasure.

Relaxation, Lubrication, and Communication

What You Should Know about
Anal Pleasure and Play

When I first started teaching human sexuality classes, the most common questions I fielded from women and men alike pertained to female orgasm, premature ejaculation, penis size, and desire discrepancies between partners. Over time, however, an increasing number of women and men began to ask me questions about anal sex and pleasuring. Whether or not they had ever engaged in these sex acts, people wanted to know more about safety and infection issues, the different kinds of anal pleasuring, and whether anal sex is common among heterosexual couples. They also regularly asked if anal sex hurt (and whether it necessarily *had* to hurt) and if there was anything that they could do to make it feel better, more pleasurable, or even orgasmic.

Though the number of people *having* anal sex didn't necessarily shift at this time, there did seem to be a cultural shift that allowed people to put aside taboos and feel comfortable thinking and asking about anal pleasure. Anal pleasuring was becoming a hot topic in many women's magazines and some newspapers. And in a research study conducted by our team at the Center for Sexual Health Promotion at Indiana University, Bloomington, we learned that women across the United States were asking questions about anal pleasure when they attended in-home sex toy parties.

Regardless of whether you choose to engage in private or partnered anal stimulation, learning more about this part of your and your partner's body can bring more relaxation, enjoyment, and connection into your sex life. But before I go into any more detail, let's take our quiz.

POP QUIZ

1. Roughly what percentage of heterosexual women and men has had anal sex?

    a. 10%
    b. 15%
    c. 25%
    d. 40%

(continued)

2. To make anal penetration more comfortable, individuals should:

> **a.** Use sufficient lubricant and go slowly and gently, stopping as needed
>
> **b.** Apply desensitizing (numbing) creams to the anal opening
>
> **c.** Thrust quickly rather than slowly
>
> **d.** None of the above—there is no way to make anal penetration comfortable for people

3. How often would you guess that people use condoms when they have anal sex?

> **a.** They use condoms *more often* for anal sex compared to vaginal sex
>
> **b.** They use condoms *less often* for anal sex compared to vaginal sex
>
> **c.** They use condoms *equally as often* for vaginal and anal sex
>
> **d.** Less than 5% of the time

4. Which of the following types of anal play are common among women and men?

> **a.** Anal massage (finger stimulation around the anal opening)
>
> **b.** Analingus (oral stimulation of the anus)
>
> **c.** Anal penetration with a finger, toy, or penis
>
> **d.** All of the above

Answers: 1) c; 2) a; 3) b; 4) d

Unlike other sexual behaviors we've discussed so far, such as vaginal sex, oral sex, and the use of sex toys, only about 15 to 25 percent of heterosexual men and women have tried anal sex.[1]

·

Of those who have tried it, not everyone enjoyed their experience or participated in anal sex again, but some did enjoy it and continued to engage in anal pleasuring. In the absence of readily available, accurate information about anal sex, many people who decide to try it often go about it in all the wrong ways. Because they haven't learned about the differences between the vagina and the anus, for example, many couples do not use lubricant when they try to have anal sex—and without lubricant, it is difficult for anal sex to feel comfortable or pleasurable (let alone for it to be safe). In addition, more people might feel open to anal play if they learned about the numerous ways of engaging in anal pleasuring, including those that have nothing to do with penile-anal sex.

The good news is that, although anal sex isn't for everybody, those who do want to give it a try can have a much easier, more comfortable, and more pleasurable experience if they learn some basic information about this part of the body and its pleasuring possibilities. After reading this chapter, I hope that you will feel:

✱ Knowledgeable about several different types of anal play, including some types that don't involve any penetration

✱ Comfortable looking at or examining your anal area without shame

✱ Able to talk to your partner about your feelings related to anal play

✱ Confident that you can explore anal play in ways that are both safe and pleasurable

✱ Comfortable talking to your healthcare provider about anal health issues

Though as many as 1 in 4 adults have tried anal at some point in their lives, many more people are curious about it or have explored other types of anal play. For example, you may have had a partner unexpectedly venture further south with their fingers or tongue, to the area around your anus, in the middle of performing oral sex. Or perhaps you have had the experience of having vaginal sex with a partner and then feeling their finger reach down to stimulate the area around your anal opening, or just inside your anus. Other times, women have considered (or tried) stimulating their partner's anus during sexual activity, whether with their tongue, finger, or a toy. This chapter is about all of these things and more, and while largely directed toward those who are new to anal play, there's also plenty of information for those of you who are seasoned in anal play, too.

WHY DOES IT MATTER?

As I mentioned at the beginning of this chapter, I firmly believe that learning about and becoming comfortable with your own and your partner's anal area can promote more pleasurable sexual experiences, even if you never try any type of anal sex play. Why? Primarily because in order to totally— and I do mean *completely*—relax and embrace the emotional and physical joys of sex, it is helpful to feel at ease with your entire body. Given how close the anal opening is to a woman's vulva and a man's penis and scrotum, becoming comfortable with the anus can facilitate comfort with other aspects of sex, such as giving or receiving oral sex. In addition (and you may have already had such an experience), it is not uncommon for women and men to experiment with anal play. You may find that one day, in the midst of an intimate moment, your partner will reach down to touch or stimulate your anal opening with their finger or tongue, perhaps unexpectedly. Perhaps you have even tried this with a partner yourself, by touching or otherwise stimulating their anal opening during vaginal intercourse or oral sex.

Perhaps because it is difficult for many women and men to talk openly about sex, some people read about anal play in a magazine and, rather than talk to their partner about it or ask for their thoughts, spring right into action. I can't tell you how many women and men I have spoken with who were surprised to feel their partner unexpectedly touch their anal opening while they were having some other type of sex. While some people are turned-on by this, others are not—they may tense up or feel anxious or unsure about what they are supposed to say or do in response. Even if a woman's partner only touches her anus for a moment and then moves on to touch another part of her body, her anxiety over this "surprise touch" can get in the way of her sexual arousal and ability to orgasm, particularly if she is worried that her partner is going to try to touch her anus again or if she feels unsure about how to respond.

HEALTH BENEFITS

Becoming more knowledgeable about this part of your body is also beneficial for your sexual health. At various times in a woman's life, she may experience anal medical issues including tiny cuts or tears (such as from straining while constipated), warts (from infection with the human papillomavirus, or HPV), or hemorrhoids—particularly during pregnancy. When you feel comfortable looking at, touching, and talking

(continued on page 162)

HOMEWORK
Getting Acquainted

Though our homework exercises usually come at the end of each chapter, in this instance, I'd like to encourage you to read through—and maybe even try—your homework assignment before reading further. This exercise is designed to help you get more comfortable with your body, whether or not you ever do anything sexual involving your anus.

The first step toward becoming comfortable with your anal area is to become familiar with it by looking at and touching it. Women who have already become comfortable looking at and touching their vulva may find this exercise easier than women who have not. Feel free to revisit the homework exercise from Chapter 2 (related to performing a vulvar self-examination and exploring vulvar touch) one or more times, until you feel at ease, before trying this exercise.

When you are feeling ready, you might begin by taking a warm shower or bath in order to relax or wind down, as well as to help you to feel that your whole body is clean, including the area around your anal opening. Many people have been raised to believe that the anus is very dirty. Although fecal matter does contain bacteria, if you are generally hygienic in your toilet and bathing practices, you are likely quite clean in the area around your anal opening. Waste is stored in the rectum, rather than the anus, and there are two muscles (the internal sphincter and the external sphincter) that close this storage area off so that waste does not pass through the anal canal until you go to the bathroom.

Once you are feeling relaxed and clean, try getting into a comfortable position that allows you to view your anal area, preferably in a well-lit room with a mirror that allows you to see enough of your body. Different people experience different feelings when they look at their anal area. Some are curious, interested, or take a "scientific" approach to their exploration. Others feel turned-on or aroused and may enjoy the sensuality of the exercise. Still, some may feel uncomfortable, ashamed, or bored. Whatever you feel is okay. Over time, just as your feelings

•

about your breasts, thighs, or abdomen may evolve, so might your feelings about your anus.

If you feel anxious, remind yourself that the anus is a normal part of the body. It may help to think about the different reasons why people look at or touch the anal opening. On a daily basis, parents look at and clean the bottoms of their babies or young children. Caretakers sometimes clean elderly patients in this area. Similarly, your gynecologist has seen and likely touched this part of your body during a quick rectal exam (see "Your Gynecological Care" on page 171), and you may have allowed other professionals to see or touch your anal area, such as during a Brazilian bikini wax or full-body checkup at the dermatologist. When it comes to sex, most people have both performed and received oral sex, which means that if there was the faintest amount of light in the room, you have likely seen your partner's anal area and he or she has likely seen yours.

The anal opening has a puckered appearance that may be similar in skin tone to the rest of your body, or it may be darker, gray, pink, or red. (The latter is true, in particular, if the skin is irritated or inflamed from constipation or hemorrhoids.) Unless you remove all of the hair in your anal and genital area through waxing, shaving, or other processes, you will likely notice some hair around your anal opening; this is normal for both women and men. If you notice bumps or lumps, you might mention them to your healthcare provider, who can give you feedback as to whether they are normal or whether they are a sign of a sexually transmissible disease (STD) or another skin or health condition. If you do see something, keep in mind that in most cases, small bumps are nothing to worry about. As you become accustomed to looking at and touching your anus, you will develop a better sense of what is normal for you, and you will be able to report any changes to your healthcare provider.

(continued)

HOMEWORK—CONTINUED

As you look at your anal area, try using gentle touch around the anal opening. You may notice that the anal opening and the area immediately surrounding it are quite sensitive; this area is rich with nerve endings, which is one reason why many people enjoy anal stimulation. Sometimes women who are curious about the sexual possibilities of anal play are disappointed if they don't immediately find it arousing to touch their anal area. If this is the case for you, try reminding yourself that this is only an exploration exercise—it is not designed to be erotic or sexually stimulating. You may experience the same types of touch as sensual or sexual when they're tried in a different context, such as when you are feeling highly turned-on, in a sexual frame of mind, and ready to explore privately or with a partner. Touching can feel very different when you are aroused, versus just sort of poking around, and you may want to explore what it feels like to be touched when you are feeling superexcited and "into it."

about your anal area, you will be better situated to notice anal symptoms, to bring them to the attention of your healthcare provider, and to apply medication, if necessary. After all, it's much easier to apply creams or ointments when you actually feel comfortable looking at the body part that needs treatment!

WHAT'S WHAT

As mentioned earlier, the anal canal is relatively short—about $1\frac{1}{2}$ inches long—and two muscles stand between it and the rectum, which is just less than 5 inches long. Other muscles are in this area, too, including the pubococcygeus muscle (also

●

known as the PC muscle, which is used during Kegel exercises; see Chapter 8). However, the two muscles that are most commonly discussed in terms of anal play are the external and internal sphincters. The external (outer) sphincter is under your *voluntary* control, meaning that you can relax and contract it at will. The internal sphincter, however, is under *involuntary* control, meaning that its muscle cells relax or contract of their own accord. Many people find that with practice and patience, they can get their body accustomed to accepting anal penetration. Some practice this by gently inserting a lubricated finger an inch or two inside their anal canal while they are taking a shower. Others build trust by having a partner insert a lubricated (and condom- or latex glove–covered) finger into their anus during sex play. When attempting anal penetration, it can help to take long breaths in and out, to aid in relaxation. For more detailed suggestions and guidelines for private or partnered practice, I recommend reading *Anal Pleasure and Health* by Jack Morin, PhD,[2] which is widely considered a classic in the field.

ANAL PLAY MUSTS

Once you have become more comfortable with and knowledgeable about your anus, the two major prerequisites for self-stimulatory anal play are **relaxation** and **lubrication.** For anal play that involves a partner, a third "must" is **communication**— hence the often-used anal play mantra of "relaxation, lubrication, and communication."

Relaxation is not only important in terms of relaxing the external anal sphincter, but as you'll recall from earlier chapters, relaxation helps to promote overall sexual arousal and ease of orgasm. It is one of the fundamentals of any form of pleasurable, enjoyable sex. Lubrication is necessary because the anus, unlike the vagina, does not lubricate on its own (see the opposite page). Silicone-based lubricants last longer than water-based lubricants, but either one may be used to promote pleasurable, satisfying anal play. (If you are using sex toys for anal play, see Chapter 6 to choose a toy-compatible lubricant.) For anal pleasuring, try using more lubricant than you initially think is necessary, keeping in mind that most people need more lube for anal penetration than they would ever consider using for vaginal sex.

Communication, while important during any sexual activity, is particularly important during anal play, as it can be more emotionally or psychologically sensitive or taboo for some people and can be more uncomfortable or painful for the receptive partner (the person whose anus is being stimulated or penetrated).

MOTIVATIONS FOR ANAL PLAY

I would also recommend that women consider why it is that they want to engage in anal play. Many women do it for the same reason that they engage in other forms of sex play: either because it feels good or because they have *heard* that it feels good and they want to find out for themselves. Some women find anal play and anal sex to be quite pleasurable, but others find it uncomfortable or painful, and you should only do what feels right to you.

In some instances, women engage in anal sex play because they believe it is "safer" than vaginal sex. This belief may contribute to the fact that women use condoms less often for anal

●

FACT: *Unlike the vagina, the anus does not lubricate on its own.*

You may remember from Chapters 2 and 4 that the vagina lubricates on its own as part of the sexual arousal process. But no matter how sexually excited or aroused a person becomes, the anus does not produce its own lubrication. As a result, anal penetration is made more comfortable and pleasurable through using a personal lubricant.

MYTH: *Anal sex hurts.*

Anal sex *doesn't have to hurt*—if it does, please stop, reassess, see if you can make it more comfortable, or give up on it for the moment. Just as about 10 to 15 percent of women find vaginal sex to be painful, preliminary research suggests that a similar proportion of individuals find that anal sex hurts too much to continue. That means, however, that a good number of women and men find anal sex to be comfortable and pleasurable. Relaxation, lubrication, and communication—as well as education about the anus and rectum—are the keys to improving and enjoying anal sex.

sex than they do when they engage in vaginal sex. However, anal sex carries significant health risks for women, including the possibility of small cuts or tears during sex. And because these cuts and tears make direct contact with the bloodstream more likely, there is an increased risk of contracting HIV and other STDs from an infected partner. However, even women with disease-free partners should take precautions against cuts or tears, as such injuries can make it uncomfortable to sit, wear certain clothing, or go to the bathroom.

That said, it is true that a woman cannot get pregnant from anal sex (unless there is "spillover" of semen into the vagina) and women who either cannot afford or cannot access birth control sometimes turn to anal sex as a way to be sexual while avoiding pregnancy risk. Other times, women feel that as long as they don't have vaginal sex, they are still virgins (in one study, 1 out of 5 women and men did not consider anal sex to be "sex"), and so they may have anal sex but not vaginal sex until they get married or otherwise find someone they want to have vaginal sex with.

Some women are interested in anal sex or other types of anal play not because it appeals to them, but because their partner is interested in trying it. If your partner's desire is what inspires you to learn about anal stimulation, and if you both find it to be pleasurable, that's wonderful. If, however, you really don't want to engage in anal sex or other types of anal play but are willing to do so because your partner pressures you to, I'd strongly suggest that you consider other ways of being sexual together. As discussed in other chapters, engaging in sex that you truly do not want to be a part of usually does not translate into pleasurable sex. In regard to anal sex, emotional discomfort or anxiety can translate into serious physical discomfort or pain, as well as a greater risk of tearing. Sometimes women worry that if they don't want to have the kind of sex their partner desires, they may be left, rejected, embarrassed, or harmed in some way. If you feel this way and have trouble saying "no" to sexual acts that you don't want to participate in with your partner, please consider connecting with a counselor or therapist who can support you in ways that promote your independence and safety.

TYPES OF ANAL PLEASURING

Just as there are many ways to pleasure a woman's vulva and vagina or a man's penis and scrotum, there are several types of anal pleasuring.

Anal massage is a common form of anal play that does not involve inserting anything into the anus; rather it is an *external* form of pleasure. Some people start by massaging their partner's buttocks and then slowly work their way closer to the anal opening. (It is similar to touching a partner's inner thighs before stimulating their genitals.) Using a water- or silicone-based lubricant to gently touch and massage the area around the anus, and the anal opening itself, can feel extremely sensuous and pleasurable and can be a gentle way of easing into anal play. Both women and men may find this enjoyable; some partners take turns with anal massage.

Analingus (also called rimming or oral-anal play) involves kissing, licking, or otherwise using one's tongue to stimulate a partner's anal opening, and possibly just inside the anal canal. Essentially, it is oral sex for the anus. Because analingus can transmit hepatitis or a range of other bacterial or viral infections, it is generally recommended that couples use a latex dental dam or a condom cut in half as a barrier between the

Anal Bleaching

Anal wha-? You heard me right: Some salons now offer anal bleaching or lightening services to lighten the skin around the anal opening. This is done purely for cosmetic reasons, as there is no health benefit to anal bleaching or lightening, and, in fact, it may cause anal irritation, discomfort, or pain. Please check with your healthcare provider before using bleaching products on your anal area.

giver's tongue and their partner's anus. You can add lubricant to the receiving partner's side of the latex (or add it directly to the anal opening) to increase their pleasure and comfort.

Anal penetration may be a part of private masturbation or couples sex play and can involve the insertion of a finger, toy, or penis. (When it involves a penis, it is most commonly referred to as "anal sex.") Again, keep in mind that the anus does not lubricate on its own, so it is important to use water- or silicone-based lubricant during anal penetration or anal sex. Many health professionals also urge people to put a condom (or latex glove, if applicable) over one's finger, toy, or penis and to then add lubricant over the condom before inserting it into a partner's anus. This can reduce the risk of cuts and tears, fingernail snags (in the case of finger play), and infection for both partners. If the person inserting their finger happens to have a cut on his or her finger, then they also risk infection via disease transmission through the bloodstream. Similarly, by wearing a condom over his penis, a man can not only protect his partner from the possibility of an STD, but he can also reduce his own risk of infection or irritation (including prostate infection, as bacteria can travel down his urethra and into his prostate).

BOOTY TOYS

If you've ever shopped for sex toys at an adult bookstore, online, or at an in-home sex toy party, you have most likely come across several types of **anal toys** (also called **booty toys**). Given the wide range of toys on the market, it is important to understand a bit about the different types so that you can choose a toy that promotes comfort, safety, and pleasure. (For information about toy materials and other safety issues, see Chapter 6.)

Butt plugs are like dildos, but for the anus. They are sometimes called anal probes or anal dildos, and while most do not vibrate, some do. A very important difference between butt plugs and vaginal dildos has to do with the base of the toy. You may remember from Chapter 2 that the vagina is only 3 to 4 inches long when unaroused and roughly 6 inches when aroused. At the far end of the vagina lies the cervix at the tiny opening to the uterus. With normal use, there is simply no way that sex toys such as vibrators and dildos are going to get past the cervix and into the uterus, as the opening is much too small. Therefore, toys used for vaginal play are always within reach and are not in danger of "getting lost."

The anus is a different story, however. Though the anal canal is short, the rectum is longer and it continues to curve into the body as it nears the large intestine—so there is a good deal of space through which a wandering sex toy can travel (or

The P-Spot

Some have nicknamed the prostate "the P-spot" in recognition of the pleasure that many men feel when it is stimulated. A man or his partner can stimulate the prostate directly by inserting a lubricated and condom- or latex glove–covered finger or sex toy into a man's anus, about 2 inches inside and in the direction of his abdomen. Like anal penetration for women, this is best done when a man is already highly aroused (possibly by using anal massage as foreplay). The prostate can also be indirectly stimulated by massaging one's knuckle into the perineum (the area on the outside of the body that lies between the scrotum and the anal opening), either as its own form of sex play or during vaginal or anal intercourse. For detailed tips and techniques related to prostate play, check out *The Good Vibrations Guide to Sex* by Cathy Winks and Anne Semans (see Resources on page 234).

"get lost," as the case may be). How might a sex toy get lost? People often get very into their sex play and how it feels to be penetrated with their toy (or another object; see "Sex Ed" on page 174), and the next thing they know, the internal sphincter may involuntarily contract, thus sucking the toy or object upward and further into their body. If you don't believe me, you should see some of the X-rays that doctors have taken of "anal foreign bodies"—objects that have become lodged so far inside the body that they had to be removed by an emergency room doctor. Believe me, this procedure is not pretty!

That doesn't mean that you cannot or should not use anal toys during sex play. It does mean, however, that you should choose a sex toy carefully. When shopping for butt plugs or anal probes, choose those that have a wide base, which can make it easier to hold onto the toy and less likely that it will get sucked up into the anus should the internal sphincter suddenly contract and draw it upward. And while covering the toy with a condom and lubricant is important, try to confine the lubricant to your anal opening and the penetrating part of the condom-covered toy, keeping the lube away from your fingers and the base of the toy. This will help you hold onto it more firmly and keep it from slipping. Though butt plugs and other anal toys can be held during stimulation, some couples find it sexy to use a **strap-on** during anal play. This is a harness worn by one partner, which holds a butt plug or dildo in place in order to penetrate the other partner. Some sophisticated strap-on models even include a vibrator on the harness so that the wearer of the strap-on can receive stimulation at the same time that he or she stimulates a partner.

Anal beads are another common toy type. A typical set is made up of a series of about five beads, usually made of soft

Your Gynecological Care

A routine part of many annual gyn exams includes having a recto-vaginal exam, during which your doctor typically inserts a finger into your rectum. This is different than a rectal exam, the purpose of which is to examine your rectum for any changes or health issues. A recto-vaginal exam, however, is another way for your doctor or nurse practitioner to feel your uterus and ovaries. As you may know, ovarian cancer is difficult to detect in its early stages, and a recto-vaginal exam can help health-care providers detect changes or abnormalities from another angle. Because of the potential to transfer the human papillomavirus (HPV) from the vagina to the anus, some experts now suggest that doctors change gloves after performing the (vaginal) pelvic exam and put on a new glove before they begin the quick recto-vaginal exam. Ask your healthcare provider about this if you have questions or would like to make sure that he or she takes this precaution. You should also let your healthcare provider know if you engage in anal play so that they can monitor you for STDs or other health risks.

plastic or silicone, that are evenly spaced along a string or a plastic or silicone band. At the end of the strand is a large ring (sometimes called the "lifesaver") that one can hold on to during insertion and removal. People typically play with beads by slowly inserting them into the anus and then slowly removing them, sometimes at the time of orgasm. Many anal bead sets are designed to be used one time only and then discarded, as they can be difficult if not impossible to clean thoroughly. Those that are linked with cotton string are impossible to clean well, whereas soft plastic or silicone beads that sit on a nonporous plastic or silicone band may be somewhat easier to clean—but I'd still recommend covering the beads with a condom before using them for anal play.

Though there are a number of anal play–related **numbing creams** (booty creams, or desensitizing creams, are also sold as gels, ointments, or liquids) available for sale, health professionals often recommend against using them. Why? Given how important your body's signals of discomfort and pain may be to alerting you to potential tearing or damage, it is important that you be able to stay aware of your body's responses and then stop, or adjust your positioning, as needed. Numbing creams can dull your ability to notice, and thus to respond, to discomfort.

TIPS AND TECHNIQUES

In addition to my earlier suggestions to use a condom and lubricant for any type of anal penetration, these additional tips can make anal penetration more comfortable and pleasurable.

✱ **Start small.** Try inserting one lubricated (and possibly condom- or latex glove–clad) finger into your own or your partner's anus before inserting anything larger (such as a toy or a penis). This can help to relax the receptive partner and ease both people into anal play.

✱ **Go slowly,** both during the insertion and during withdrawal. Deeper thrusting and a quicker pace can cause discomfort or pain, so go easy and talk to each other so you can both understand how the other is feeling and whether you want to keep going or stop.

✱ **Stop if it hurts.** Anal penetration does not have to hurt. Not even a little bit. If it hurts, stop. You can always try again later (or never).

✳ **Go smooth.** Anal toys should be smooth, without any sharp edges. Nails should be carefully filed (and again, fingers are best when covered with a condom or a latex glove).

✳ **Stay sober.** Given the risk for tearing and infection, anal penetration is best approached when you and your partner are not intoxicated or using drugs. If you feel like you need to get tipsy in order to have anal sex, try spending more time getting comfortable with each other's bodies, or indulge in extra sessions of anal massage and other nonpenetrative anal play before trying anal sex. If you can't talk about it and relax enough on your own, you're probably not ready to try it yet. If you are ready, stay sober during the act and celebrate with a glass of wine afterwards.

✳ **Don't cross-contaminate.** The vagina is quite sensitive, so please do not stick anything (fingers, a toy, a penis) into the vagina after it has been inside the anus. If you are (wisely) using condoms, then use a new condom each time you have vaginal sex and another new condom for anal sex.

✳ **Keep breathing!** Just like working out at the gym, it is important to keep breathing. When you breathe in and out, you promote relaxation, which can make anal play more comfortable.

✳ **Use dedicated toys.** For the ultimate in good hygiene, dedicate a certain toy for vaginal play and another for anal play, and don't get them confused. Toys are affordable enough these days that there is no reason to use the same two toys in both places, thereby risking vaginal irritation or infection.

POSITIONS

Thanks to images from porn, when people think about anal sex between a woman and a man, they often imagine a woman on all fours being penetrated from behind by a man—and possibly with a good deal of thrusting and some choice, condescending words. No wonder many woman are wary of anal sex!

Like every other form of sex, though, if you are interested in trying it, it is up to you to approach it in a way that feels right to you. A colleague once told me that he thought more women would find anal sex pleasurable if they tried it from a position that gave them more control over their own bodies and the angle of penetration. As such, you might try woman-on-top or other positions that you enjoy when having vaginal intercourse. The positions are the same, the only difference is that penetration involves the anus rather than the vagina. Others prefer missionary, but with the woman's hips raised on a pillow, to facilitate her relaxation and access to her anal area.

The rectum, in addition to being longer than the vaginal

Sex Ed

Medical literature is full of reports of patients who have "lost" various items in their rectum through unsafe anal play. As such, let me remind you that you should never use objects for anal play that have the potential to get lodged inside your anus—nor should you ever use items for anal play that have sharp or rough edges or chemicals that might irritate the delicate rectal tissue. And if you're curious about some of the things emergency room doctors have had to remove, the list includes carrots, zucchini, shampoo bottles, beer bottles, plastic cups, and broom handles![3]

canal, is curved toward one's tailbone. Because of its curved shape, many people find that, when trying anal penetration or anal sex, it helps to experiment with different postures and positions to find one that they can feel relaxed in and thereby experience penetration with ease. Specifically, it helps to angle one's finger, toy, or penis toward the tailbone, following the curve (see the diagram below), so as to work with the shape of the rectum rather than against it.

DO WOMEN ORGASM THIS WAY?

Although some women orgasm during anal sex, it isn't always the anal stimulation that sends them over the edge. Many women stimulate their clitoris with fingers or a vibrator while they are enjoying anal play, and others enjoy both vaginal and anal penetration at the same time (sometimes called "double penetration," or "DP" for short). Similarly, although some

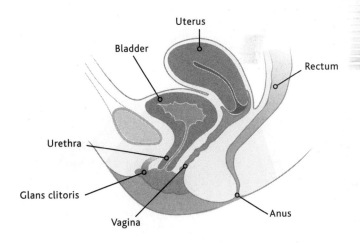

men orgasm when they are the ones being anally penetrated, they often stimulate their penis at the same time, too. Anal pleasuring is often a complement to an existing sexual repertoire.

As far as what people like about anal play, that varies. Because the anal opening is rich with nerve endings, many women and men like how it feels to have the area touched, massaged, or penetrated. For some, the pleasures may be more psychological in nature and related to the sense that anal play feels forbidden or erotic. Men who enjoy receiving anal stimulation also get the added bonus of having their prostate stimulated (see "The P-Spot" on page 169).

Positions and Techniques

Tips, Tricks, and Why
Missionary Is Underrated

Now that we've covered the basics of anatomy, arousal, desire, orgasm, and toys, let's take your new sexual knowledge and confidence a bit further and look at how you can enhance your experiences of self-pleasuring and partner sex. Because this chapter is packed with tips, I invite you to think of it as a resource that you can come back to time and again to try something new or to consider a fresh approach to something that's become familiar. Sexual tips and techniques have different meanings and applications for different people. For instance, right now you might want to learn a new position as a way to increase your odds of having an orgasm; in a month or a year, you may find that you're newly curious about using toys or

●

spicing up your self-pleasuring. This chapter can serve as an evergreen resource, no matter what drives your desire to change things up. Ready to begin?

POP QUIZ

1. Which position may help women orgasm?

    a. Woman-on-top

    b. Rear entry

    c. Side entry (scissors position)

    d. Coital Alignment Technique

2. The most sensitive parts of a woman's breasts are the:

    a. Tops

    b. Sides

    c. Nipples

    d. Areolas

3. Which Eastern practice has been shown in studies to possibly boost women's sexual function?

    a. Reciting a mantra

    b. Transcendental meditation

    c. Mindfulness

    d. Fasting

4. Women who find it easier to orgasm during oral sex tend to worry less about the way that their genitals:

    a. Look

    b. Smell

    c. Taste

    d. All of the above

Answers: 1) d; 2) a; 3) c; 4) d

As you can see from this chapter's quiz, I think about tips and techniques in different ways than other sex experts might. My experience working with women and men has underscored the importance of both the mind and body in sexual pleasure. People can twist themselves into the most creative sexual positions or try highly sophisticated sexual techniques, but if they are not feeling relaxed, open to pleasure, or present in the moment, they are unlikely to find that sex feels good. My goals in this chapter are to help you:

* Understand the importance of a holistic, mind-body approach to sexual pleasure

* Feel confident that you can apply mindfulness practice to sex

* Be able to identify areas of your own or your partner's body that may be more sensitive or pleasurable when stimulated

* Feel comfortable exploring your own or your partner's body in pleasure-focused ways

* Learn how to adapt sexual positions in ways that feel more comfortable, enjoyable, and potentially orgasmic

OPENING YOURSELF TO PLEASURABLE SEX

Perhaps the most important step you can take on your path to feel-good sex is to open yourself to a wider range of pleasure possibilities than you may have initially imagined you'd enjoy. *Of course I'm open to pleasure*, you might be thinking. *That's why I'm reading this book!*

Hear me out, though.

In my experience, many women and men could benefit from opening their minds and imaginations a little bit more than they already do. Historically speaking, sexual information has been kept a secret from women in particular (and men, too), so the fact that many women and men are now in touch with their bodies and sexual responses is exceptional and exciting. Many people can now confidently say that they know what they like—and they may indeed know the easiest, quickest way for them to have an orgasm and the position, fantasy, or vibrator that works the best for them.

I want to suggest, however, that although sometimes the "easiest, quickest" path to pleasure or orgasm is the one to choose, more often than not I would encourage women and men to think about sex in a different way.

IT'S THE JOURNEY, NOT THE DESTINATION

Allow me to illustrate this point: Think about a place, such as your office, your child's school, or a grocery store, that's located at least 5 to 10 minutes away by car and that you go to regularly. Have one in mind? Okay, now think about how you would normally get there from your home. My guess is that you know the quickest route or the one with the fewest traffic lights or stop signs. But do you know every possible route between point A and point B? Unless you live on the next block, probably not. Do you know three or four different scenic routes that will get you there? Or the route that has particularly breathtaking views at sunrise or during a full moon? What about the route that takes you by luscious gardens or landscaped homes, or a pond laid claim to by a flock of Canada geese? Perhaps there's even a route that takes you by a park where, if you pass it at just the right time, you might catch a glimpse of children playing tag or men and women practicing tai chi.

This is a helpful way to think about the process of opening our minds to sex: We may be missing adventures and beauty when we only seek the fastest, most reliably orgasmic route. In our quest to have the "best sex ever," do we risk missing out on a rich variety of experiences of "really, really good" sex? Of course it makes sense to do what you know will feel good, but not if it means sacrificing the chance to experience a little bit of

Genital Self-Image and Cunnilingus

In 2005, I surveyed more than 400 female college and graduate students and found that women who found it difficult to orgasm during cunnilingus tended to worry about their genital taste, smell, appearance, and whether their partner was enjoying themselves. Not only did they feel anxiety about their own genitals, but they also tended to hold a less-positive view of women's genitals in general (compared to women who found it easy to orgasm during oral sex). Having surveyed more than 200 men, too, I learned that men generally felt very positively about women's genitals—how they looked, smelled, and tasted—and rather than dreading going "down there," most men reported that they enjoyed performing oral sex!

If you think oral sex is something that you might like but you feel hesitant about trying it, remember: Relaxing into sex, staying in the present, and reframing negative thoughts into positive ones (turning "I hope I don't smell too bad" into "This is so hot, and it feels so good") can help to make cunnilingus—like other sex acts—feel good inside and out. Also, keep in mind that you don't have to stick with it for the long haul; you can try it briefly and move on to other activities, if you want.

chemistry or magic, or the opportunity to really relate to a person you like, love, or feel safe with.

First and foremost, then, I'd like to encourage you to let go of certainty and to imagine that there may be two, five, or fifty ways that you can enjoy sexual intimacy. Just as our preferences for foods, drinks, partners, and friends change throughout life, so might our sources of sexual pleasure. You may feel some resistance toward seeing yourself in this more ambiguous way. At times, you may think, "But I *like* doggie style! Why should I do missionary?" Of course you can always return to your favorite position, but I am asking you to replace a negative, knee-jerk reaction at the thought of trying something new with positive, explorative, open thoughts, like "I may find missionary to be erotic and arousing."

It makes perfect sense for individuals and couples to explore their own and each other's bodies and to develop a repertoire of sexual behaviors or whispered words that make them feel good. I'm simply suggesting that, every now and then, it's a good idea to explore other ways of being intimate.

SEX WITH INTENTION

It is often said that a person's biggest or most important sex organ is their brain. Time and again, research supports the fact that the brain plays an important, influential role in our sexual response. The mind-body connection has a real impact on the way we experience sex.

Both women and men are susceptible to what are sometimes called "cognitive distractions"—thoughts that can pop into your mind during sex and keep a person from feeling immersed in the sexual experience. These thoughts can be about anything at all—work, school, arguments, family stress, body issues, or even something as silly as a television show you watched earlier. If you find that you predictably get distracted at certain times or in certain situations, make note of that. You might try planning your sex around those instances. For example, if after your weekly dose of *Lost* or *24* you find yourself becoming distracted during sex, record the show and watch it another

Three Tips for Better Fellatio

1. **REINVENT IT.** Some women dislike performing fellatio because they have a sense that there is only one way to give a guy a blow job, and that's gaggingly deep and all the way through to orgasm. Men who dislike it often feel that way for similar reasons—except for them, it may feel like pressure to perform or to have an orgasm. Remember: Your sex life is your own and you can reinvent it in any way that you like. Don't want to go deep? Stick to licking the shaft or head. Don't want to swallow? You don't have to. If you'd rather use it as foreplay or an intermission, rather than the main event, please do! Your partner may thank you.

2. **EMBRACE ENTHUSIASM.** Time and again, men describe enthusiasm—a sense that their partner is excited about and savoring the experience—as a key contributor to pleasurable fellatio. Which makes sense: Think about how you feel when your partner suddenly, passionately kisses you, compared to when he gives you an obligatory good-bye or goodnight kiss. One is way hotter than the other.

3. **ENJOY VARIETY.** Many roads lead to Rome, so consider licking or exhaling warm breath on the head; kissing, stroking, and licking the shaft; licking the scrotum; trying different paces (slow and sultry versus fast and feverish); and stimulating his perineum with your knuckle, fingers, or tongue. (See Resources on page 234 for detailed fellatio guidebooks.)

time or, if you really want to have sex that evening, try having sex before the show begins.

Though there are multiple strategies to address distractions, one of the most innovative methods now being used to help women tune into their sexual arousal is mindfulness. Mindfulness training has been shown in studies to help women access their arousal more easily, feel more sexually satisfied, and feel free to enjoy sex.[1] In one of these studies, although the participants had taken part in an intensive program that also involved relationship skill-building, therapy, and pelvic floor muscle strengthening (think Kegels), they rated the mindfulness training as the most helpful component of the program.

Mindfulness is the practice and experience of being present in the moment. Many prominent Buddhists have advocated the idea of bringing mindfulness practice into everyday life, as it has been shown to reduce stress and anxiety, improve sleep, and promote happiness.[2] Mindfulness can also enhance sexuality. It makes sense—if you consider the more pleasurable moments of sexuality that you've experienced, you likely felt completely engaged and "into" the moment, thinking only about yourself and your partner. You probably weren't trying to remember the name of the place where you had dinner last week or reminding yourself to call your sister later.

Being mindful and engaged in the present can help women and men focus on the pleasurable sensations experienced by their bodies. Noticing that your sexual response is, in effect, "in working order," can be particularly reassuring for those who have thought that their ability to become aroused or to respond sexually had disappeared. Mindfulness is also a way of focusing your attention, and it can help you avoid getting pulled into distracting, distressing, or negative thoughts.

●

BECOMING MINDFUL

Begin by practicing brief (5- to 10-minute), daily mindfulness sessions to help you learn how to still your mind and fully experience the present. Try starting off with the exercise below. While it only takes a moment to read, allow yourself at least 5 minutes to complete it. You'll probably find that the more you practice, the easier it will get. If you are interested in learning more about mindfulness, there are many books and CDs available that can teach you how to develop this practice in depth (see Resources on page 234).

Begin by getting into a comfortable position and closing your eyes. Notice how your chest and stomach feel as you breathe in and then out in an even rhythm. Focus your attention now on the way that your thighs feel on the chair or pillow that you're sitting on, and how your feet feel on the floor. Listen for any sounds that are around you, and focus your attention on them for a few moments. Then notice any scents in the air for another minute or so. Consider, too, the temperature and how you are holding your body and your face. What feels tense, and which parts respond to deep breaths and efforts at relaxation?

You can also try this exercise with your eyes open, or while taking a bath and feeling warm water enveloping your body and warming your skin. You can progress from there to focus on mindfulness while walking, eating, or even exercising. You may come to find that you enjoy these activities even more than you did previously.

Applying mindfulness to situations in your everyday life can be a comfortable way to practice and become familiar with this method of thinking and feeling. Once you bring your mindfulness practice into the bedroom, you may begin to notice more tingly or warm sensations in your genital area, or

Sex Ed

A word about pace: Though vigorous sex is often passionate and exciting, slow sex can feel more seductive, pleasurable, or orgasmic for some women. Try keeping yourself open to—and curious about—the possibilities of sexual variety.

pleasurable feelings elsewhere in your body. Or you may notice the way your breathing effects your sensations. Pay attention to how your different body parts feel, to the weight of your partner's body against yours, and to the sights, sounds, scents, and touches that feel good.

SEXUAL MINDSET

Try to foster a sexual mindset that helps to focus your arousal. What do you find erotic? What makes you feel tingly all over? Allow your mind to drift and explore, from subtle turn-ons you may not have considered before to your wildest fantasies. Refer back to Chapter 4 to learn more about cuing arousal through activities such as reading erotic stories, viewing sexual materials, thinking about an exciting sexual experience from your past, or thinking about what you might enjoy doing with an imaginary lover—or your real one! It's okay if it takes time to get into a sexual mindset; foreplay, mindfulness, and relaxation can all help you get—and stay—there.

SQUEEZE, RELEASE, REPEAT: THE JOYS OF KEGELS

Kegel (KEY-gull) exercises are performed by squeezing and then releasing one's pelvic floor muscles, also called the pubococcygeus muscles or "PC" muscles. They're named after Dr. Arnold Kegel, a physician who identified the relationship between weak pelvic floor muscles and incontinence and sexual problems. Though many women are familiar with Kegel exercises as a treatment for incontinence, performing Kegel exercises has also been shown to improve sexual function. This is particularly true for women who are dealing with incontinence issues, which can make them feel hesitant or uncomfortable with their sexual response. In fact, a 2003 study published in the *International Urogynecology Journal*[3] found that women with incontinence who were trained in pelvic floor exercises noticed increases in both desire and ease of orgasm.

Even women who are not struggling with incontinence may benefit from performing Kegel exercises, as may men, given that Kegels have been shown to help premature ejaculation and erectile problems, too. Kegel exercises are performed in numerous ways. The first key is to identify one's PC muscles, which can be done by contracting the pelvic floor muscles as if you were stopping the flow of urine. It's a subtle contraction and you can't tell just by looking at someone whether or not they are doing Kegels, which means that you can practice them just about anywhere! Think about practicing while stopped at a traffic light, changing a diaper, sitting in class, or working at a desk. Different Kegel "routines" are sometimes recommended by sexual health professionals. Some examples include:

* 10 quick, forceful contractions followed by 10 slower contractions that last 5 to 10 seconds each

* 5 minutes of many rapid contractions

* 20 contractions and releases, lasting 3 to 5 seconds per contraction and 3 to 5 seconds per release

To keep things interesting, you might vary the pace, rhythm, or force that you use when you practice for about 5 minutes or more per day. If you have a partner, you might even try doing your exercises together on occasion, for quirky but potentially fun foreplay. If you're specifically using Kegels to respond to incontinence, or if your male partner is using them as a way to address premature ejaculation or erectile dysfunction concerns, I encourage you to also check in with a healthcare provider to rule out the possibility of other health issues.

Aside from potentially boosting sexual function for some women and men, Kegel exercises have another sexual enhancement function: They may simply feel good! Some women find that squeezing their PC muscles feels arousing, and they use these movements to get themselves in the mood for sex or to enhance vaginal lubrication. Also, some women find that Kegels are fun to use during intercourse—and many men enjoy the feeling of having their penis squeezed during vaginal sex. Try using different paces to contract your PC muscles while in missionary or rear entry. If you're on top, try squatting over your partner, rising up (while still engaged in intercourse), and then squeezing along at different points of his shaft or head for varied sensations and pleasure, both his and your own.

SENSATIONAL SENSATION

Moving away from the genitals for a moment, let's hear it for the rest of our bodies! Though vulvas and penises are fabulous works of art (and pleasure), they make up a small percentage of our bodies, not to mention our pleasure systems. Our bodies

FACT: *There is no one "best" condom.*

Although many women and men have personal condom preferences, condoms that are sold in the United States have to pass certain safety tests in order to be cleared by the U.S. Food and Drug Administration. Most but not all condoms that are sold overseas would meet the same criteria. If you're traveling abroad, consider packing your own condoms or purchasing brands and styles that are familiar to you (even if that fact that they're "imported" makes them more expensive).

MYTH: *A lubricant is a lubricant is a lubricant.*

Not so. Because lubricants are not regulated in the same way that condoms are, and because little research has been conducted on them, it is unclear which lubricants may be best for whom. Some healthcare providers suggest that women and men with diabetes might want to steer clear of flavored lubricants, given the sugar content; others recommend that women who are prone to yeast infections should avoid lubricants that contain glycerin. Similarly, some women and men are sensitive to ingredients such as propylene glycol or chlorhexidine. Always check the label to see what ingredients your lubricant contains.

Finally, couples who are trying to become pregnant might consider skipping the lubricant, as some research suggests that common lubricants may impair fertility, perhaps by altering the pH of the vagina or decreasing sperm's motility. That said, recent studies have found that some lubricants (such as Pre-Seed and ConceivEase) may be more "fertility-friendly" than others.[4]

are covered with skin that responds to touches, kisses, and licks, and I'd be remiss to skip over our other important parts. Here are a few quick briefs on women's and men's bodies.

BREASTS

✱ A woman's breasts are actually most sensitive on the tops and bottoms, then the sides, and finally on the areolae and nipples—information that's surprising to many people. If you like breast play, encourage your partner to start on the outside and work his way in, focusing on the nipple last—if at all—and see what types of touch feel good during your own self-pleasuring. (See the photo on the opposite page.)

✱ Just because breasts are sensitive does not mean that you want to have them touched. This may be particularly true for women who are going through hormonal changes (which can cause breast soreness or tenderness) or who have babies or young children to care for and who may feel as though their breasts are always being touched. It is okay to want a break from breast touching and to express that to your partner.

✱ Speaking of breasts, larger breasts (C and D cups) tend to be less sensitive than smaller breasts; this may at least partly explain why some women enjoy breast play and others don't. Sensitivity also tends to decrease with breast augmentation (implants) and increase with reduction.

✱ Nipple balms and even some lip balms can create tingling sensations that may make your breast play and kissing more fun—not to mention tastier for the licker.

✱ A woman's breasts, when smooshed together, can do more than create cleavage. If you have a male partner, try putting his penis between your breasts for sex play—

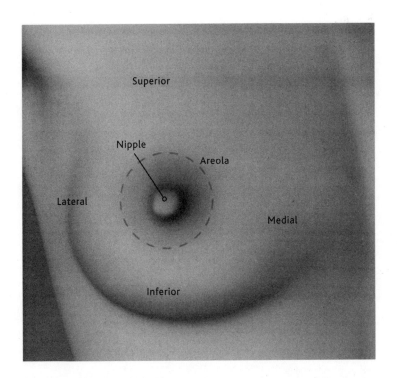

some women find that this is particularly pleasurable during foreplay and can make performing oral sex easier or at least different.

THE REST

* The inner thighs can provide a lovely stopping point on the way to one's genitals. Use your hands to touch or mouth to kiss or lick the thighs prior to, or during, oral sex.

* Fingers and hands need love, too. Remember when you were younger and first starting to hold hands and maybe—just maybe—kiss? A crush's hand reaching for

•

yours could send shivers down your spine! Don't let cobwebs settle—hold your partner's hands, kiss their hands (or your own—seriously, it may make you remember what you're missing!), or suck on a partner's fingers as an oral sex teaser.

✻ Back and neck massages remain a prime foreplay technique, given how partners can use this time to relax, practice mindfulness, and slip into a sexual mindset. Try spending considerable time massaging each other in ways that promote both relaxation and sensuality.

ON HIM

✻ On the underside of a man's penis, the frenulum (the triangular area just below the glans; see opposite page) may be particularly sensitive and responsive to delicate touch or licks.

✻ His testicles like attention, too—during oral sex, try licking or sucking (gently) on a testicle and see how he likes it.

✻ The "P-spot" (prostate) can be accessed from inside or outside of a man's body—some men prefer internal stimulation with a lubricated finger (use a latex glove or a condom over a finger, for safer sex) or toy inserted in the anus. Other men may prefer to be stimulated externally at the perineum with a knuckle. If you're unsure whether a man will enjoy anal pleasuring, ask before trying, as comfort levels vary. To learn more about anal pleasuring and prostate stimulation, see Chapter 6.

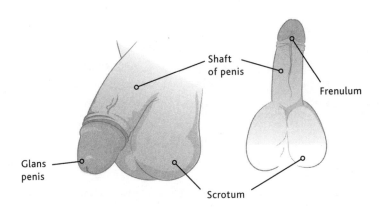

Shaft
of penis

Frenulum

Glans
penis

Scrotum

DIY SEX

Masturbation is the ultimate do-it-yourself experience that most women and men have tried at some point in their lives. Also called self-pleasuring, it usually involves the genitals but may involve other types of body touching or no touching at all—just fantasy.

Keep in mind that—as with partner sex—relaxation, mindfulness, and a sexual mindset can ease your experience of genital arousal and orgasm. Some women find it helpful to set a scene that encourages relaxation and a deeper sensual experience, such as lighting scented candles, taking a warm bath, or dimming the bedroom light.

Sex Ed

If a vibrator feels too intense, put a soft cloth or towel between your body and the vibrator, turn the intensity down (if it has multiple speeds), or use it over your clothes or underwear.

To enhance your masturbation, try varying your technique from time to time.

✳ Consider using a lubricant during masturbation. Research conducted by our team at the Center for Sexual Health Promotion at Indiana University, Bloomington, suggests that women may find masturbation and partner sex more pleasurable when they use a water- or silicone-based lubricant.

✳ During masturbation with a dildo or vaginal vibrator, try propping your hips up on a pillow so as to tilt them upward or downward, and see how that changes your vaginal sensation. You can create a similar effect by varying the angle of penetration with a dildo.

✳ Take a bath! Women who discovered their genital sensitivity while taking a bath will tell you how marvelous, soothing, or even ticklish it can feel to let warm (not hot!) water drip on one's genitals.

Signature Move: The Hip Tilt

Mum's the word as to where this came from, but suffice it to say that during vaginal intercourse, you might be surprised by what a little hip tilt can do. During missionary, try keeping your hips tilted upward at a 30- to 45-degree angle. After maintaining this for some time, quickly (and without warning) tilt your hips downward. Bonus points if you simultaneously squeeze your PC muscles. The sudden shift in stimulation can feel pleasurable to a partner, and it may help to trigger his orgasm. (So careful, then, if you're depending on the not-so-reliable method of withdrawal as birth control!)

✱ Have phone sex with your partner. Just because you're in different time zones (or simply living across town) doesn't mean you can't be together. Put your phone on speaker or use an earpiece for maximum comfort and to free up your hands for self-pleasuring.

G-SPOT EXPLORATION

One of the most common methods of exploring the G-spot to find out what feels good is to use two fingers in a come-hither motion or a similarly shaped dildo or vibrator to stimulate the front wall of the vagina. (See Chapter 2 for a G-spot primer and below for an example.)

That said, if you are exploring your G-spot privately or with a partner, a few tips might make your play more pleasurable.

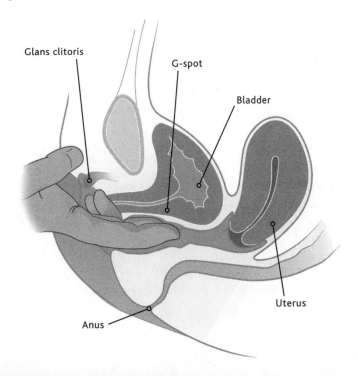

Glans clitoris

G-spot

Bladder

Uterus

Anus

First, remember that the G-spot isn't necessarily all that it's cracked up to be. Though many women find stimulation of the front vaginal wall to feel pleasurable, not all do. When you're feeling relaxed, aroused, and lubricated, allow your own or your partner's fingers, a toy, or your partner's penis inside to stimulate the front wall (the same side as the belly button), just an inch or two inside. If you're using your fingers, you may feel a raised bump or an area textured like a walnut shell. Or you may feel neither texture, but still think it feels good!

Remember, gentle but firm pressure tends to encourage G-spot pleasure more so than light tickling stimulation does. Because G-spot stimulation likely stimulates the internal clitoral branches (the crura), the erectile tissue surrounding the urethra, or both, some women find that "sandwiching" the front vaginal wall can intensify their pleasure. Try this by stimulating the vagina gently but firmly with a finger, toy, or penis, as well as by externally— and simultaneously—pressing your hand firmly but gently on your mons pubis (the triangular area at the top of your genitals). Lying on one's stomach during G-spot exploration can provide similar stimulation.

POSITIONS

More often than not, pleasure and orgasm are in the details when it comes to positions. Thus, in the pursuit of feel-good sex, there's no need to master the full range of *Kama Sutra* positions—but a little curiosity (what would it feel like if I tilted my hips like this, squeezed harder, or slowed it down like that?) can go a long way.

I believe that **missionary position** is enormously under-rated. It is perhaps the most commonly used position in most cultures and it sets us humans apart from many animal species in that it allows for face-to-face contact, thus facilitating the emotional side of a sexual experience. Perhaps the best—and most scientifically tested—variation on missionary is the **Coital Alignment Technique** (CAT; see the image on page 198), which has been found to help women have orgasms during inter-course. Like traditional missionary, the woman lies down and her partner is on top, but he positions his body further along her body (with his shoulders closer to her head and shoulders). Her knees are typically slightly bent at less than a 45-degree

Sex with a Latex Allergy

Got a latex allergy? So does 1 to 6 percent of the general population and about 10 percent of healthcare workers (thanks to regular exposure to latex-containing equipment, such as latex gloves). Follow these tips to reduce your risk of an outbreak caused by sex.

* Choose polyurethane condoms.

* Be careful with sex toys: Even those described as "silicone" are often silicone-based, and that "base" may contain latex. Opt for toys that you're sure are latex-free, such as glass dildos or hard plastic toys; slip a polyurethane condom over a toy if you're not certain.

* Use nonlatex gloves for safer finger or hand stimulation of the vagina or anus.

* Try to keep sex on the bed rather than getting into it on the floor, as some carpeting may contain latex, according to the Centers for Disease Control and Prevention.

* For safer cunnilingus, use a polyurethane condom cut in half, rather than a latex dental dam.

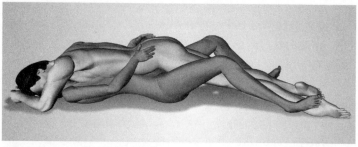

Coital Alignment Technique (CAT)

angle. The main focus, rather than on male thrusting, is
on pelvic grinding and rocking to enhance both clitoral and
G-spot stimulation.

In more traditional versions of missionary, in which
partners' bodies have more space between them, a silver bullet
or finger vibrator can be used for clitoral stimulation during
intercourse.

Woman-on-top (WOT) is often cited as a position that helps
women orgasm more easily. Orgasmic or not, WOT is pleasurable for many couples. This can be true for several reasons:
Women who experience discomfort or pain during intercourse,
or who have a particularly well-endowed partner, may find that
being able to control the depth of penetration and the pace of
intercourse makes for a more comfortable and pleasurable
sexual experience. Other women find that WOT makes it easier
to zero in on G-spot stimulation, such as by leaning backward
while on top, thus pressing the front of the vaginal wall against
a partner's penis.

Also in WOT, a woman might rise up and withdraw her
partner from her body for a slow **massaging variation** in which
she leans back on her forearms and slowly, sensuously slides
her vulva up and down her partner's shaft, which can feel
pleasurable—and look sexy—for both partners.

A **squatting variation** involves sitting with one's knees up and "bouncing" on (or slowly sliding up and down) a man's penis (see below). Men who otherwise find it difficult to maintain their erection during WOT may find that the sliding stimulation in this modification is helpful. Take care, though, as a penis can be injured during sex in any position in which it comes out and then accidentally "pops" against a partner's body while headed back in. If this happens and your partner is in pain, he should seek medical treatment.

A woman can use a **masturbation sleeve** with two openings by sliding it over her partner's penis and then sitting on top. This is a particularly useful variation for women who have a partner with a penis that is long enough to feel uncomfortable during sex. Incorporating a sleeve into intercourse gives his

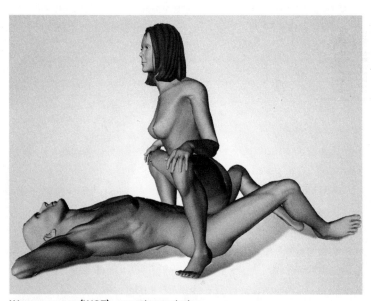

Woman on top (WOT), squatting variation

HOMEWORK
Sex Lessons

If you feel open to the idea of trying something new or unexpected, consider trying a Sex Lesson on for size. This can be done by yourself or with a partner. Here's how:

> **Privately:** Choose a time during which you are unlikely to be interrupted, and use it to find out what your sensual and sexual responses can teach you about your body. Some women find that they like to try this in a bathtub; others feel more relaxed in bed. Begin by breathing deeply and finding a place of calm. Using your hands, begin by touching your inner wrists, forearms, or thighs, noting how it feels for them to be touched with long, slow, gentle, almost ticklish strokes. Now change the touch to shorter or deeper strokes and note any differences in feel. Move on to another part: You might massage your scalp, rub your shoulders, gently play with your hair, touch the spaces between your toes, circle your breasts with your fingers (using lotion or not), or touch different parts of your vulva. Again, note how your body feels; do you feel warm or tingly in any places? Has your heartbeat slowed or quickened in response to a certain type or placement of touch?

penis more stimulation along its length while giving the woman less to take into her body.

In **rear entry**, a woman may find that changing the angle of her torso can alter sensation: Like deep thrusting? Try supporting yourself on all fours, back straight like a table. For less depth and more hair-pulling (hey, some people like it!), rise up from all fours onto your knees, or arch your back intensely. Craving shallow thrusts and slow grinding? Start on all fours,

Which of these touches turn you on or encourage you to feel
interested in sex?

With a partner: Sex Lessons with partners can be playful and
offer the opportunity for you to learn about each other's bodies
and turn-ons. Each person should have at least 10 to 20 minutes
to explore the other person's body without interruption. Only
when that person has had their full time should they either move
on to another sexual (or nonsexual) activity or trade turns with
the other partner. You can ask for verbal feedback (such as "that
feels good," or "try a slower touch there") or nonverbal feedback,
like moans for pleasure or a shake of the head for things that don't
feel good. I favor verbal feedback because I think it is clearer,
though if you and your partner are new to communicating about
sex and bodies, nonverbal feedback may be more comfortable for
you. Make sure to spend time on body parts other than the genitals and, when you do touch and explore the genitals, try to do so
in new ways. Use this exercise as a way to develop communication about likes and pleasures.

then slowly sink into the bed (bodies practically melded
together) until you are lying on your stomach, with your partner
lying on top. (This is very good for G-spot stimulation.)

Rear entry is also well-suited to using a couple's vibrator,
such as the We-Vibe, as during missionary it may uncomfortably press against a woman's pubic bone. Rear entry allows a
woman the space to press it against her clitoris while still
enjoying its use for vaginal stimulation. As a bonus, the

•

We-Vibe can also be removed from the vagina and gently held around the base of a man's penis for partner masturbation play—after all, many men like vibration, too! (Remember: Always clean toys and make sure you are both STD-free before sharing toys with a partner.)

In yet another variation on rear entry, a woman can stand next to the bed, bending over with her stomach and chest on the bed. Depending on her height, she may find that bending her knees slightly helps to press her mons against the corner of the bed, which, as described earlier, can heighten sensation on the front wall (G-spot area) of the vagina.

Talking about Sex

Improving Communication within and beyond the Bedroom

Just because love, attraction, and sexual chemistry may, at times, feel magical does not mean that they have to feel mysterious. Our personal, romantic, and sexual relationships are too important to keep in the dark, particularly given that healthy relationships are critical not only to our happiness but also to the stability of our families and communities. Learning communication and relationship skills can enhance our sex lives and bring a level of clarity and contentment to our committed relationships.

This chapter is meant to provide you with specific strategies that you can use to communicate about your body, your sexuality, and your relationship. Even though many women and men have taken part in short-lived flings or casual affairs, the vast majority of people's sexual experiences tend to take place within the context of a relationship. Considering that numerous studies have linked good sex to healthy, satisfying relationships,[1] it makes sense for people who are interested in sex to also pay attention to their relationships. I'm not suggesting that there's such a thing as a "perfect" relationship. However, we can all improve our relationships by learning to talk to each other with respect, kindness, and appreciation so that we can have the sex—and love—that we want and deserve. Ready to begin?

POP QUIZ

1. What percentage of married adults are largely satisfied with their sexual partner?

    a. 54%
    b. 64%
    c. 84%
    d. 94%

2. Women's lust for their partner is linked to:

    a. Feeling satisfied with their partner
    b. Feeling happy with their partner
    c. Their partner's level of lust
    d. All of the above

3. Which of the following is true about marital satisfaction?

    a. It tends to increase after a couple has a baby together
    b. It tends to decrease after a couple has a baby together
    c. It is usually not affected after a couple has a baby together

4. What percentage of women and men feel preoccupied with their sexual performance?

    a. 5% of women, 10% of men

    b. 15% of women, 15% of men

    c. 30% of women, 50% of men

    d. 50% of women, 50% of men

Answers: 1) d; 2) d; 3) b; 4) c

Many women and men grew up in families that did not talk about sex or that spoke about it in ways that were not helpful. You may have heard sex talked about in ways that suggested that women who had sex outside of marriage or who dressed in revealing clothes were "tramps" or "sluts," or that men "only wanted sex" (rather than love). Some people recall hearing their families or friends make mean or hurtful comments about women or men because of their sexual orientation; others remember being told that they were "bad" or "dirty" for touching their genitals, or for making out with a boyfriend or girlfriend. These messages can make it difficult for people to figure out how to talk about sex with their partner, particularly if they feel too embarrassed or ashamed to say sexual words (such as clitoris, orgasm, vagina, or semen) out loud; if they don't yet feel comfortable asking to be touched in a certain way; or if they're not at ease telling their partner how often, or how rarely, they would ideally like to have sex—and why.

If you're uncomfortable talking about sex, it can cause more than relationship problems. Countless studies have documented the fact that doctors and nurses often don't ask patients about their sexual health, or they may not warn patients that certain medications, surgical procedures, or health conditions may have sexual side effects, simply because they are too embarrassed or worried that their patients will feel embarrassed.[2] Ironically, many patients have the same concerns about discussing sexual health issues with their healthcare providers.

Learning to communicate effectively about sex can enhance your romantic relationship and your overall sexual health. As such, my goals for this chapter are that when you're done reading it you will begin to be able to:

* Talk about sexuality in a way that feels more comfortable than embarrassing

* Express your wants, needs, likes, dislikes, and curiosities to a partner

* Effectively listen to your partner's wants, needs, likes, dislikes, and curiosities

* Move beyond feelings of awkwardness to talk to your healthcare provider about your sexual health

DO WE REALLY HAVE TO TALK?

When couples first get together, their sexual chemistry and mutual interests may be enough to keep them feeling satisfied with their relationship and their sex life. However, as discussed in earlier chapters, couples, and especially women, tend to need more from their relationship in order to feel interested in and excited about sex as a relationship progresses. Many women feel as though talking is a form of foreplay and a way for them to feel closer to their partner. In fact, people who feel emotionally

●

close with their partner are more likely to experience increased sexual satisfaction and desire.[3]

Talking is important for other reasons, too. When sexual problems occur—and the vast majority of couples will be confronted with at least one sexual difficulty if they stay together long enough—communicating with one another can help a couple move beyond the problem and find a solution.

Healthy sexual communication is particularly critical when a couple's life shifts in a dramatic way, such as when they start a family. Numerous studies have shown that relationship satisfaction tends to be lower among couples who have babies or young children.[4] While children are one of the greatest joys in many people's lives, there is no doubt that having a child changes the way that partners relate to one another, including the amount of free time that they have for sex.

THE EBB AND FLOW OF LUST

If you have ever been in a long-term relationship or marriage, or if you are in one now, then you likely know that feelings of love and lust ebb and flow. Sometimes you may feel crazy about your partner, and at other times you may feel less excited. This is true for both feelings of love and feelings of sexual passion.

In 2006, researchers from the University of Arizona published a fascinating study in which they asked couples to track their feelings for each other every day—including their levels of lust—for a period of about 2 months.[5] As you can imagine, they found very different patterns from person to person. Some individuals rarely felt much passion or excitement for their partners, whereas others experienced high desire one day and low desire the next. Every participant experienced ebb and flow

Girl Talk

Although learning how to talk to your romantic partner is important, so is talking to your girlfriends! In fact, many sexuality experts believe that we could all greatly benefit from learning how to talk, joke, laugh, play, and support not only the other gender, but those of our same gender, too. In some ways, men are better at this than women are, or at least they seem to have more opportunities to meet friends. For example, a man who is new to a school or a town can literally walk up to a bunch of complete strangers on a basketball court and join in on a game of pick-up. Except for the small window of time during which women have young children whom they take to playgrounds or nursery school, women have fewer opportunities to make friends with other women.

This can take its toll on your romantic relationship. After all, no human being (man or woman) can be "everything" to their partner—nor should they be. We are all enriched by being able to express different parts of ourselves with different people. You may have a partner who helps you to feel safe, calm, and secure, but also cherish your best friend who can make you laugh until your stomach hurts. There may be movies or musical events that greatly interest you but bore your partner. Why not catch them with a friend?

Try to look for ways to connect with other women in your community, whether through your child's Parent Teacher Association (PTA), the Junior League (a women's volunteer, philanthropic, and leadership organization that has roots in many towns internationally), your place of worship, or a local volunteer agency whose work you admire. On the Web, check out CheekyChicago.com, which started in Chicago in 2008 (but is now expanding to other cities) as a way of connecting women with their communities and with each other through an online community and local events that encourage female bonding over food, fashion, the arts, and more.

•

in their level of passion. After all, not even the happiest couples "always" feel enormous chemistry for one another. We all get sick, stressed, or irritated sometimes.

The findings from the research study also confirmed what others have found in previous studies: Members of a couple were more likely to feel lust for each other on days when they generally had positive feelings (contentment, satisfaction, happiness) about each other and had few negative feelings (anger, irritation, anxiety, neglect, sadness) for each other. And when a participant's other half was high on passion, they were more likely to feel that way, too. Lust was also linked to feelings of closeness and equality in the relationship. The more that you can learn to talk, listen, empathize, and state your needs, the more likely you are to feel satisfied in your relationship and embrace the passion that is available to you. Here's how you can begin to do that.

GET TALKING NOW—
BEFORE PROBLEMS START (OR GET WORSE)

I frequently ask men and women whether they talk to their partner about sex when they are not having, or about to have, sex. For instance, do they discuss their sex lives while sitting on the couch (completely clothed) or driving in the car? Depending on the group I'm talking to, as many as 95 percent of the people in the room have said that they *never or only rarely* have such conversations. This response is common even among couples who have been married for 20 or 30 years. And yet your partner is exactly the person you should be talking to about your sex life, as he or she has the power and possibility of working with you to make it better!

It's a good idea to share your likes, dislikes, concerns, fantasies, or hopes with one another outside of the bedroom, when you're not engaged in an intimate moment. That way, even if difficult feelings come up, you won't feel increased pressure to perform or run the risk of ruining a particularly sexy moment. I highly recommend that you practice talking to your partner about sex so that you feel more comfortable initiating a conversation. Try the following:

✳ **Identify a time when you two can talk—uninterrupted.** Try to find a time and place in which you are unlikely to be interrupted by a favorite TV show, sports event, children, work, or your own fatigue. For some couples, their private talk time occurs in the bathtub. (Angelina Jolie has gone on record saying that this is when she and Brad Pitt like to talk.) For others, it is while driving in the car to or from work, or while lying in bed on weekend mornings. Choose what works for you.

✳ **Be clear.** When you have something specific that you'd like to talk about, let your partner know. For example, say that you would like to talk about your sex life. (Because this book is about sex, we'll stick to that; but you can use this time to talk about other relationship issues, too.)

✳ **Be gentle.** University of Washington researcher and relationship expert John Gottman, PhD, has found that the way couples begin a conversation matters. If you want to bring up a difficult issue, try what he calls a "softened start-up." For example, rather than saying "I hate how you make me feel bad when I don't want to have sex," try "I really want our sex life to get back on track, and I feel

like I could use some support from you in figuring out
how to do that."

✶ **Move past the awkwardness.** When you first try to talk
about sex with someone, or you try again after a difficult
past, it can feel awkward to allow yourself to be
vulnerable. That's okay—take deep breaths and go with it.
With time and practice, sex talks usually become more
comfortable for both partners.

✶ **Find words that work.** A unique challenge related to
talking about sex is that people don't always know what
words to use, or they may not feel comfortable saying or
hearing certain words. There are emotionally charged
choices to be made when choosing words for body parts,
such as vulva/genitals/pussy, penis/dick/cock, as well as
sex acts themselves, such as making love/having sex/
fucking/doing it. Some women and men are open to a
range of words; others have particular preferences. If all

Hearing Things You Don't Like

Let's face it—when you start communicating with honesty, you
sometimes hear things that you don't like. You may learn that your
partner doesn't enjoy the way that you touch him, or that your favorite
sexual position is his least favorite. (Oops—that look in his eyes turned
out to be irritation rather than excitement!) On the bright side—and
there truly is a bright side here—when you know what your partner
doesn't like, you are actually in a great position because now you can *do*
something about it. You can take a hit, acknowledge the hurt, and move
on to brainstorm together about how to make your sex life better. It is
okay to say, "That was hard for me to hear, but I understand. How can
we work together to improve this part of our sex life?"

sexual words make you uncomfortable, practice saying them out loud or reading books like this one to help you become comfortable with a limited vocabulary. You may find it helpful to let your partner know what your boundaries are in terms of which words you prefer. Some couples even invent their own special words for their genitals or for sex acts.

✳ **Pay attention to the positives.** The vast majority of women and men—94 percent, in one study[6]—said that they were satisfied with their sexual partner. And yet a lack of communication leaves many women and men wondering how their partner feels about them. Use these conversations as opportunities to discuss the fun and joyful parts of sex as well as the areas that need improvement. Telling your partner something that you liked about a past sexual experience you shared provides valuable feedback about how you like to be touched or pleasured. Lavishing compliments can also help to cushion the times when you need to say something difficult. Examples of sex compliments include: "The other night was really special to me; I liked how you took the time to give me a massage before we made love," or "I can't believe I had an orgasm in that one position last week—that's never happened before! I appreciate how patient you are with me."

✳ **Start now.** It's wise to practice your sexual communication before problems begin or get worse. If conflict has already escalated to a painful, hurtful level, you may find it helpful to meet with a counselor or therapist who can support you both through the process of trying to repair your relationship.

SEX NOISES (AND CONVERSATION)

One of the more common sex questions (and frustrations) that men, in particular, have about women is that they often wonder why so many women are completely quiet, or almost nonresponsive, during sex. If this describes you, you might ask yourself what contributes to your silence. Are you worried about looking or sounding aggressive, silly, or out of control? People generally enjoy seeing their partner let down their guard during sex—it is, after all, an incredibly natural experience of pleasure. Why not embrace it whole-heartedly? Moans and groans, or saying "more," "over here," or "yes, there," can be extremely helpful as your partner tries to pleasure you.

If your partner makes pleasure noises or talks during sex and you do not, your silence may be intimidating. Sometimes people wonder if their partner's silence indicates distraction or a lack of enjoyment. It is perfectly fine to be quiet during sex if that is how you feel most comfortable, though if that's the case, you may want to find ways to reassure your partner of your feelings about your relationship and sex life.

If you would like to try to be a little more vocal during sex, start slowly with the occasional moan in response to a touch or thrust that feels good. Some women find that it is easier for them to experiment with noises while they are getting a professional massage. It is common for massage clients to make noises of relaxation (such as sighs of release or moans of relaxation), and sometimes it is easier to let go in front of a stranger than one's own partner.

Noises aren't the only possibility—you can also talk to each other during sex. Some couples share fantasies or recall other highly arousing sexual times that they've had ("I'm thinking about that time on vacation when I got on my knees and went down on you, and then we had sex on the balcony. . . ."). Other times, talking is brief and related to what's happening in the here and now, as in "What would you like to do next?" or "Can I get on top?" Keep in mind, too, that sex can go on for as long as you have time for. Some child-free couples, empty nesters, or vacationing partners make sex quite a main event. They may spend two or three hours talking, kissing, sharing a bath, drinking wine, having sex, talking some more, having more sex, and so on. Talking can be intertwined throughout sex, making it one of several enriching, connecting experiences.

POST-SEX TALKS

One of my favorite ways to encourage women and their partners to talk about sex is to suggest they try a post-sex play-by-play (rather than have them "just roll over and turn out the light" like the unhappy couple in the Neil Diamond/Barbara Streisand duet "You Don't Bring Me Flowers"). What's a post-sex play-by-play? If you've ever watched a football game, you've certainly noticed the play-by-plays, during which the announcers describe what certain players did, what worked,

Relationship Guru

Learning to improve communication is easy for some couples and quite challenging for others, especially if they have been locked in hurtful patterns for many years. If you would like to direct more dedicated attention to your relationship dynamics, allow me to suggest pretty much any book written by Dr. John Gottman, a man who has spent his career at the University of Washington studying and trying to understand the characteristics that help couples to succeed as well as those that put them at risk for trouble. See Resources on page 234 for suggestions of particularly helpful titles.

what didn't, who scored, and so on. In a post-sex play-by-play, you and your partner "review" the sex that you just had. Keep the conversation light-hearted—it's supposed to be fun!—and full of compliments and kindness. Save the tough stuff for your special sofa, car, or bathtub talk. A post-sex play-by-play might look something like this:

(Following sufficient cuddle time and the chance to bask in feelings of closeness or a post-orgasmic glow)

WOMAN: *I really liked that move you did with your tongue. That was new.*

HER PARTNER: *What move?*

WOMAN: *The one where you went in circles and then zeroed in on my clitoris. It felt really good—I would definitely like to try that again.*

HER PARTNER: *Good to know! I like pleasuring you like that. It's hot.*

WOMAN: *Thanks. I like it too. What did you think about me being on top, and moving slowly? I know you often like it faster but going slow felt really good at the time for me. How did it feel for you?*

HER PARTNER: *It was good. I liked it. I definitely like it when sex is fast, too, probably because it's easier for me to stay hard. But slow was good, too; I like how deep it felt when we were going slowly.*

With post-sex play-by-plays, you both have a chance to review what just happened and to give (and get) immediate feedback, rather than having to wait to catch up another time (or risk forgetting to compliment each other altogether). Plus, if either one of you had a particularly strong emotional response

●

in terms of feeling distant, sad, tearfully joyous, or highly connected, you can talk about that, too, and clear up any misunderstandings. For example, if—during sex—you suddenly felt very distracted because you started thinking about work, then you have a chance to tell your partner that if you seemed distracted, here's why. Play-by-plays can help couples to affirm the good parts of their sex life while simultaneously clearing up any misunderstandings.

EFFECTIVE LISTENING

As important as it is for romantic partners to talk to each other, good communication requires that they *listen* to each other, too. Because people often say that they are listening when they are only doing so half-heartedly, therapists and educators often use the term "effective listening" to describe a more conscious, thoughtful form of listening. It generally involves the following:

✳ **Giving full attention.** In a 2007 study, attention and involvement (meaning eliminating outside distractions and setting up private time to talk) were two of the most effective strategies that women and men used to build closeness.[7] Try turning off the television, closing the newspaper, and abandoning the computer while you listen to your partner, child, or a family member. It communicates to that person that they are valuable and important to you, and it allows you to devote your full attention to the conversation.

✳ **Taking turns.** When your partner is talking, it is your turn to listen carefully. If you find yourself thinking about what you want to say next or about reasons why your partner is wrong and you are right, then you are not doing the work that listening requires. Preparing to win an argument or a debate suggests that you may be missing out on a chance to understand the other person's perspective.

✱ **Listening for feelings.** Often, especially when someone is very upset or nervous, they may not choose the best words. They may say things like "You never kiss me when you come home" when what they mean—if you look for the embedded feelings—is that they wish they were kissed more often, or that they crave affection or love from you. Focusing on the feelings can help direct you to the more vital issues.

✱ **Having empathy.** It can feel difficult, even painful, to talk openly about relationship struggles—especially sexual ones. One study found that 30 percent of women—and about 50 percent of men—felt that they were often preoccupied with their sexual performance.[8] Men often feel enormous pressure to perform sexually, which can increase as they age and become more vulnerable to erection, desire, and prostate problems. Try to express your empathy for your partner and the hurt, embarrassment, or frustration that they might be feeling. Have some empathy for yourself, too. Relationships take a lot of work, and they make people vulnerable to each other in striking ways. Know that sexual issues are a shared problem that you can get through together.

✱ **Clarifying the need.** In our "can-do" culture, we often try to jump in and fix things for our partner or friends. If someone is complaining to you, wait until there is a break in the conversation, then consider asking if they want to vent their frustrations or if they are looking for advice or information. Sometimes jumping in too quickly to fix things can make matters worse, and it can feel good for the person who is venting to feel listened to, even if no solution is in sight.

✻ **Showing that you understand.** Try to use validating statements, such as "I can understand why you're so frustrated" or "Anyone would feel hurt." You might even paraphrase your partner (loosely) to make certain that you've understood correctly. For example, you might say "I get it—it makes you feel bad when I tease you about erection problems." Letting your partner know that they have been heard is a crucial part of communication.

SHOW AND TELL

While it is true that couples can learn a great deal from talking and listening, they also learn by doing. Women, and especially men, tend to believe that they should somehow know how to please their partner. The truth is, we all have to learn, and most people learn about sex from their friends, books or magazines, or movies. If you work on your communication, you and your partner can gain an enormous amount of sexual knowledge about one another.

A couple's sex life can be enriched through grown-up versions of "show-and-tell." Generally, this involves asking your partner to show you how they like to do something (or you volunteering to show your partner how you like to do something). For example:

FACT: *Communicating about sex is good for your health!*

Even if your healthcare provider does not ask you about your sexual health, I want to strongly encourage you to tell them whatever you think may be relevant (and then some—they can filter out what's not helpful). Let your healthcare provider know if you have been sexually active since the last time he or she has seen you, whether you have been sexually assaulted or are currently being physically or sexually abused, and any history that you or your partner(s) may have regarding sexually transmissible diseases (STDs), including HIV. Also, clue him or her in on any problems you may be having with arousal, lubrication, desire, genital pain, or orgasm. Some problems are linked to medications; others can be caused or made worse by health conditions or treatments, and it may be to your benefit to speak up.

MYTH: *You should be able to tell your friends anything.*

While it is nice to know that you could potentially tell your friends anything, some things are better kept private. Because everyone has a different comfort level when it comes to revealing personal information, especially about sex, check in with your partner to learn where his or her boundaries lie. He might be fine with you talking about the fun parts of your sex life, but embarrassed if you talk about his erection problems or penis size. Other times, partners don't set specific "you can say this, but not that" limits on each other, but they trust one another to make careful choices. Telling your best friend about your fertility struggles is one thing; telling the office gossip is another. Try to respect the privacy of your relationship, while still allowing yourself to share and commiserate with friends.

* How you like to use a vibrator or other sex toy

* How your partner likes to have his penis or scrotum touched

* How much lubricant your partner usually uses on his penis when he masturbates

* How gently or firmly you would like to be touched on your breasts or vulva

* Where on your vulva you most enjoy being touched

If you find yourself describing how you like to be touched, try to include a show-and-tell component by saying "like this . . . " and demonstrating for your partner. If your partner tells you about something that they like sexually, ask for them to show you. You might then take a turn doing that same thing and asking for feedback, such as by asking "How did that feel?" or "Was that soft enough?" or "Was that wet enough?" This is particularly important considering that there is no one way to have any type of sex. There are endless variations on foreplay, breast touching, vaginal intercourse, oral sex, and anal pleasuring, and the most valuable information about techniques that feel good will come from your partner.

COMMUNICATING LOVE, AFFECTION, AND DESIRE

Women and their partners can benefit greatly from finding ways to communicate and express their feelings of love, affection, and desire. Look at the list below and consider which steps might work for you—and then commit to trying at least one new thing this week. If you don't have a partner at the moment, browse the list to see which of these you could try (or modify for use) with a family member or friend. Getting into good relationship-building habits now can pay off later in a romantic relationship and can improve your friendships and family relationships, too.

✷ **Touch your partner.** Remember: Even nonsexual touch can encourage a person's body to release oxytocin, which is associated with feelings of bonding and closeness. Try out different types of touch that might work for you: a reassuring hand on your partner's shoulder, holding hands while taking a walk, laying your head to rest on your partner's chest, or rubbing one another's feet while sitting on the couch.

✷ **Say thank you.** Appreciation is vital for sustaining a loving connection with your partner. It only takes seconds to thank your partner for emptying the dishwasher, starting a pot of coffee, bringing in the mail, or kissing you in a way that makes you feel incredibly safe and secure.

✷ **Try new things together.** Research suggests that couples who try new things together experience improvement and satisfaction in their relationships in ways that spending quality time together (but doing the same old routine) does not.[9] Consider this an excuse to learn a foreign language together, go camping for the first time, try indoor rock climbing, or explore a local park that you haven't been to before.

✳ **Say "I love you" every way that you know how.** Leave a love note on the inside of your partner's laptop or in the sole of his or her shoe. Or take advantage of technology by texting a romantic message or sending a photo of a beautiful sunrise that you saw on your way to work and wanted to share. For some people, it is easier to express emotion through e-mail, IMing, and social networking sites such as Facebook and MySpace than it is in person. You have to start somewhere!

✳ **Get creative.** Explore your opportunities for expressing desire and excitement—draw hearts on the shell of a hard-boiled egg and leave it on the kitchen counter in place of a love note; draw a big heart or a sexy message on the bathroom mirror's steamy surface; lay out your partner's morning cereal and coffee mug with a quickly drawn note or picture; or make pancakes shaped like hearts (or private parts!).

✳ **Make passes at each other.** Look at your partner in sexy ways. When you can, kiss for longer or deeper than you normally do. Pull him closer and with passion. Touch or kiss your partner's genitals when it's least expected. And if you're feeling excited, it's okay to say it! Even if your partner has to rush off to a morning meeting, why not say, "I wish you could come back to bed" if that's what you're feeling? Or invite your other half to join you in the shower—though it's a tight fit, there is often room for two.

Taking steps toward bringing sensuality or romance into your life can feel daunting if this is new to you (or if it has been a while). Keep in mind that any issues you are facing in your relationship are perhaps better viewed as a shared problem rather than as something bad that only one of you has done. Shared problems need solutions for which *both* people are responsible. As such, you might show this list to your partner and say "I'd like to see more of this in our relationship—how do you feel about it?" Or you could tell your partner that you've been thinking about ways to add more romance and spark to your relationship or sex life, and you have some ideas, but you're also wondering what he or she might come up with or would feel comfortable trying.

HOMEWORK

Recognizing Emotional Bids

While we've all heard about never going to bed angry, what about never leaving your partner hungry for affection or emotional connection? Dr. John Gottman has written extensively about the notion that we all make what he calls "bids" for attention, affection, or connection. Even when we may believe that a partner, friend, or family member doesn't notice or care about us, the reality may be that we have simply not opened our eyes to the way that they bid for our attention or show us affection.

Try to expand your perspective and consider how your partner or another loved one may be trying to get you to engage with them. For example:

✳ Perhaps your partner calls you frequently throughout the day and, because you're trying to get things done, you're short or grumpy in response. His phone calls may be his way of showing love or affection. If you truly cannot talk at the moment, rather than being short, try saying "I love that you called but I'm swamped right now and feeling stressed. Can I call you back later?"

✳ You just found out that your partner signed you up for a couple's fantasy football league. You can't imagine anything less romantic, but it may be an attempt to include you in his or her world or turn you on to something fun. If you can see it that way, you may find it enriches your relationship.

✳ You feel as though your partner doesn't help out enough around the house. You do everything; he does nothing. Except that if you looked more closely you might find that he always has a pot of coffee going first thing in the morning and never uses your favorite mug. Many people—when they look more carefully—find that their partner does the little things for them, and those little things may help you to feel happier and more satisfied in your life together.

Consider your own relationship and how those around you bid for attention, affection, or connection. They might:

✳ Send you links to news articles that they think you'll find interesting

✳ Put a hand on your knee

✳ Call or text you during the workday

✳ Buy your favorite type of orange juice

✳ Get up with the children so that you can sleep in

✳ Stock up on your preferred cereal

✳ Pick up your prescriptions at the pharmacy

✳ Fill up the gas tank so you don't have to

✳ Try to make conversation or small talk, even if it's just about the weather

Think of your partner, best friend, or a family member who you sometimes feel disconnected from or neglected by. Are there ways in which he or she may be trying to connect? How might you be able to respond differently to meet him or her halfway?

Conclusion

Beginning Again

The title of this section is neither a mistake nor a typo; though we've arrived at the end of the book, for many of you this reflects a new beginning. If you have read *Because It Feels Good* because you're interested in the possibility of change for yourself or your relationship, you may feel a little overwhelmed by all the new ideas and information. You may be thinking about new steps to take or new perspectives that you can try to adapt. You may feel excited, uncertain, inspired, nervous, or encouraged as you ponder what is possible for your sex life. New beginnings can feel both fun *and* uncomfortable. It's kind of like a first date, when you're simultaneously excited by the possibilities and nervous about what might happen.

I invite you to sit with these feelings for some time, whether that is a few hours, days, or weeks. Change takes time and preparing for it can be helped by a good deal of thoughtful reflection. Try to be patient with yourself, and enjoy where you are right now. You may find it valuable to identify one or two key areas in which you would like to begin to change, knowing that

●

it is sometimes easier to successfully transform one area at a time than it is to change several all at once.

Some women find it helpful to keep a journal. Begin by writing where you feel you are in the present moment and in what ways you would like to adjust your sexual life or relationship over time. Writing down these ideas and feelings gives you a chance to make sure that you won't forget your goals as you move forward. It also provides a written record to which you can return periodically and recognize your successes, as well as the ways in which your goals may change over time.

If you and your partner are working together to enhance your shared sexual life, you might occasionally check in with one another to see how each of you is feeling about your experiences and any sexual activities you may be trying together. Change is a developmental process, and occasionally you may feel as though you are in different places. At times, one of you may feel more ready to adjust certain aspects of your life together, and the other may seem resistant. These differences occur during the natural ebbs and flows of a relationship.

Reading through this book, you may have found yourself interested in learning more about a specific topic. No book can cover everything and, as an author and someone who enjoys helping people learn about their sexual lives, I certainly wish that I had the space to cover more issues in depth. Fortunately, there are many good books that focus specifically on sexuality as it relates to subjects such as pregnancy, aging, illness, parenting, same-sex relationships, and menopause. There are also very helpful books that provide information about sexual techniques. In the Resources (see page 234), I've listed the titles of books that I often recommend to others and believe that you will find helpful, too. If you are interested in seeking professional help, you'll also find a list of organizations that

•

can help you locate doctors and therapists in your area.

As you make changes in your sexual life, try to be gentle with yourself. Take time to appreciate the ways in which you are opening your mind and heart to enhancing your relationship and your sexual life. Acknowledge the attention that you are directing toward the development of empathy for yourself and your partner, knowing that as much as you may try to please each other, emotionally or physically, there are times when you are likely to feel disappointed. That is part of being human and it happens in all relationships. There is a great deal to be gained from picking yourselves up and trying again. Along the way, remember to compliment one another's growth, express compassion, and reach out for support as needed.

As you might expect from someone who writes a book titled *Because It Feels Good,* I also hope that you will take to heart the importance of pleasure and enjoyment in your intimate life. Too often people feel pressured to be sexual in ways that they are not comfortable with, either to please a partner or to feel "normal" in society. Though sex doesn't always feel good, and I understand that, I do hope that you will consider ways in which it might more often feel good, as well as ways in which your relationship as a whole might be enhanced.

When they embark on the journey of enhancing their sexual lives, some women feel intimidated by how much there is to learn about sex and relationships. It may take time for the ideas of pleasure, worth, and dignity to seep in and feel as though they are a part of you. That's okay. The good news is that there is time enough for new beginnings. Whatever your path, you now have an enormous number of tools and resources available to you to begin to transform your personal sexual life and relationship. I wish you only the best.

Endnotes

CHAPTER 1

1 Muller, Charla, and Betsy Thorpe. *365 Nights: A Memoir of Intimacy.* (New York: Berkley Trade, 2008).

2 Birnbaum, G. E. "The Meaning of Heterosexual Intercourse among Women with Female Orgasmic Disorder." *Archives of Sexual Behavior* 32, no. 1 (2003): 61–71.

CHAPTER 2

1 D. Herbenick. "The Development and Validation of a Scale to Measure College Students' Attitudes Toward Women's Genitals." Dissertation, Indiana University, 2006.

2 Alfred C. Kinsey, Wardell B. Pomeroy, Clyde E. Martin, and Paul H. Gebhard. *Sexual Behavior in the Human Female.* (Philadelphia: W.B. Saunders, 1953).

3 P. B. Pendergrass, C. A. Reeves, M. W. Belovicz, et al. "The Shape and Dimensions of the Human Vagina as Seen in Three-Dimensional Vinyl Polysiloxane Casts." *Gynecologic and Obstetric Investigation* 42, no. 3 (1996): 178–82.

4 R. Raz, B. Chazan, and M. Dan. "Cranberry Juice and Urinary Tract Infection." *Clinical Infectious Diseases* 38, May 15 (2004): 1413–19.

CHAPTER 4

1 J. Bancroft, J. Loftus, and J. S. Long. "Distress about Sex: A National Survey of Women in Heterosexual Relationships." *Archives of Sexual Behavior* 32, no. 3 (2003): 193–208.

2 S. W. Kuffel, and J. R. Heiman. "Effects of Depressive Symptoms and Experimentally Adopted Schemas on Sexual Arousal and Affect in Sexually Healthy Women." *Archives of Sexual Behavior* 35, no. 2 (2006): 163–77.

3 C. A. Graham, S. A. Sanders, R. Milhausen, and K. McBride. "Turning On and Turning Off: A Focus Group Study of the Factors That Affect Women's Sexual Arousal." *Archives of Sexual Behavior* 33, no. 6 (2004): 527–38.

4 L. D. Hamilton, E. A. Fogle, and C.M. Meston. "The Roles of Testosterone and Alpha-Amylase in Exercise-Induced Sexual Arousal in Women." *Journal of Sexual Medicine* 5, no. 4 (2008): 845–53.

5 C. B. Harte and C. M. Meston. "The Inhibitory Effects of Nicotine on Physiological Sexual Arousal in Nonsmoking Women: Results from a Randomized, Double-Blind, Placebo-Controlled, Cross-Over Trial." *Journal of Sexual Medicine* 5, no. 5 (2008): 1184–97.

6 D. M. Ferguson, G. S. Singh, C. P. Steidle, J. S. Alexander, M. K. Weihmiller, and M. G. Crosby. "Randomized, Placebo-Controlled, Double Blind, Crossover Design Trial of the Efficacy and Safety of Zestra for Women in Women with and without Female Sexual Arousal Disorder." *Journal of Sex and Marital Therapy* 29, no. 1 (2003): 33–44.

CHAPTER 5

1 S. Brody and T. Kruger, "The Post-Orgasmic Prolactin Release Following Intercourse Is Greater Than Following Masturbation and Suggests Greater Satiety," *Biological Psychology* 71, no. 3 (2006): 312–15.

2 M. Lancel, S. Kromer, and I. D. Neumann, "Intracerebral Oxytocin Modulates Sleep-Wake Behavior in Male Rats," *Regulatory Peptides* 114, no. 2–3 (2003): 145–52.

3 S. Freud, *New Introductory Lectures on Psycho-Analysis* (London: The Hogarth Press and the Institute of Psycho-Analysis, 1933).

4 A. C. Kinsey, W. B. Pomeroy, C. E. Martin, and P. H. Gebhard, *Sexual Behavior in the Human Female* (Bloomington, IN: Indiana University Press, 1998).

5 A. Ladas, B. Whipple, and J. Perry, *The G Spot: And Other Recent Discoveries About Human Sexuality* (New York: Holt Paperbacks, 2005).

6 G. Greer, *The Female Eunuch* (New York: Bantam, 1972).

7 A. Ingelman-Sundberg, "The Anterior Vaginal Wall as an Organ for the Transmission of Active Forces to the Urethra and Clitoris," *International Urogynecology Journal and Pelvic Floor Dysfunction* 8, no. 1 (1997): 50–51.

8 C. M. Meston, R. J. Levin, M. L. Sipski, E. M. Hull, and J. R. Heiman. "Women's Orgasm." *Annual Review of Sex Research* 15 (2004): 173–257.

9 S. Ortigue, S. T. Grafton, and F. Bianchi-Demicheli, "Correlation Between Insula Activation and Self-Reported Quality of Orgasm in Women," *NeuroImage* 37, no. 2 (2007): 551–60.

10 R. V. Haning, S. L. O'Keefe, E. J. Randall, M. J. Kommer, E. Baker, and R. Wilson, "Intimacy, Orgasm Likelihood, and Conflict Predict Sexual Satisfaction in Heterosexual Male and Female Respondents," *Journal of Sex and Marital Therapy* 33, no. 2 (2007): 93–113.

11 J. Harris, L. F. Cherkas, B. S. Kato, J. Heiman, and T. D. Spector, "Normal Variations in Personality are Associated with Coital Orgasmic Infrequency in Heterosexual Women: A Population-Based Study," *Journal of Sexual Medicine* 5, no. 5 (2008): 1177–83.

12 K. Dawood, K. Kirk, J. M. Bailey, P. W. Andrews, and N. G. Martin, "Genetic and Environmental Influences on the Frequency of Orgasm in Women," *Twin Research and Human Genetics* 8, no. 1 (2005): 27–33; K. M. Dunn, L. F. Cherkas, and T. D. Spector, "Genetic Influences on Variation in Female Orgasmic Function: A Twin Study," *Biology Letters* 1, no. 3 (2005): 260–63.

13 J. Heiman and J. LoPiccolo, *Becoming Orgasmic: A Sexual and Personal Growth Program for Women.* (New York: Fireside, 1987).

14 H. De Graaf and J. Rademakers, "Sexual Development of Prepubertal Children," *Journal of Psychology & Human Sexuality* 18, no. 1 (2006): 1–22.

CHAPTER 6

1 R. Maines, *The Technology of Orgasm: "Hysteria", the Vibrator, and Women's Sexual Satisfaction.* (Baltimore: The Johns Hopkins University Press, 2001).

2 D. Herbenick, M. Reece, S. Sanders, D. Fortenberry, B. Dodge, and A. Ghassemi, "Vibrators, Sexual Health and Well-Being, and Sexual Pleasure: Findings from a Nationally Representative Sample of U.S. Adults," presented at the 136th Annual Meeting of the American Public Health Association. San Diego, CA, October 2008.

3 B. Dodson, *Sex for One: The Joy of Selfloving* 1974; reprint, (New York: Three Rivers Press, 1996).

4 C. Winks and A. Semans, *The Good Vibrations Guide to Sex* (San Francisco: Cleis Press, 1997).

CHAPTER 7

1 R. O. De Visser, A. M. A. Smith, C. E. Rissel, J. Richters, and A. E. Grulich, "Heterosexual Experience and Recent Heterosexual Encounters Among a Representative Sample of Adults," *Australian and New Zealand Journal of Public Health* 27, no. 2 (2003): 146–54; J. I. Baldwin and J. D. Baldwin, "Heterosexual Anal Sex: An Understudied, High-Risk Sexual Behavior," *Archives of Sexual Behavior* 29, no. 4 (2000): 357–73; N. E. MacDonald, G. A. Wells, W. A. Fisher, W. K. Warren, M. A. King, J. A. Doherty, and W. R. Bowie, "High-Risk STD/HIV Behavior among College Students," *Journal of the American Medical Association* 263, no. 23 (1990): 3155–3159; D. T. Halperin, "Heterosexual Anal Intercourse: Prevalence, Cultural Factors, and HIV Infection and Other Health Risks, Part 1," *AIDS Patient Care and STDs* 13, no. 12 (1999): 717–30.

2 J. Morin, *Anal Pleasure and Health: A Guide for Men and Women* (San Francisco: Down There Press, 1998).

3 D. L. Clarke, I. Buccimazza, F. A. Anderson, and S. R. Thomson, "Colorectal Foreign Bodies," *Colorectal Disease* 7, no. 1 (2005): 98–103; S. Feigelson, D. Maun, D. Silverberg, and T. Menes, "Removal of a Large Spherical Foreign Object from the Rectum Using an Obstetric Vacuum Device: A Case Report," *The American Surgeon* 73, no. 3 (2007): 304–06.

CHAPTER 8

1 L. A. Brotto and J. H. Heiman, "Mindfulness in Sex Therapy: Applications for Women with Sexual Difficulties Following Gynecologic Cancer," *Sexual and Relationship Therapy* 22, no. 1 (2007): 3–11; K. A. Mayland, "The Impact of Practicing Mindfulness Meditation on Women's Sexual Lives," unpublished doctoral thesis, California School of Professional Psychology, 2005.

2 K. W. Brown and R. M. Ryan, "The Benefits of Being Present: Mindfulness and Its Role in Psychological Well-Being," *Journal of Personality and Social Psychology* 84, no. 4 (2003): 822–48; K. W. Brown and T. Kasser, "Are Psychological and Ecological Well-Being Compatible? The Role of Values, Mindfulness, and Lifestyle," *Social Indicators Research* 74, no. 2 (2005): 349–68; K. A. Coffey and M. Hartman, "Mechanisms of Action in the Inverse Relationship between Mindfulness and Psychological Distress," *Complementary Health Practice Review* 13, no. 2 (2008): 79–91; J. E. Smith, J. Richardson, C. Hoffman, and K. Pilkington, "Mindfulness-Based Stress Reduction as Supportive Therapy in Cancer Care: Systematic Review," *Journal of Advanced Nursing* 52, no. 3 (2005): 315–27.

3 N. K. Beji, O. Yalcin, and H. A. Erkan, "The Effect of Pelvic Floor Training on Sexual Function of Treated Patients," *International Urogynecological Journal* 14, no. 4 (2003): 234–38.

4 A. Argawal, F. Deepinder, M. Cocuzza, R. A. Short, and D. P. Evenson, "Effect of Vaginal Lubricants of Sperm Motility and Chromatin Integrity: A Prospective Comparative Study," *Fertility and Sterility* 89, no. 2 (2008): 375–79; W. H. Kutteh, B. Collins, R. W. Ke, and L. J. Williams, "Conceivease Fertility-Friendly Lubricant Is Superior to Other Commercial Lubricants in Preserving Sperm Motility and Sperm Progressive Motility Over 72 Hours," *Fertility and Sterility* 90, no. S1 (2007): S324.

CHAPTER 9

1 E. S. Byers, "Relationship Satisfaction and Sexual Satisfaction: A Longitudinal Study of Individuals in Long-Term Relationships," *Journal of Sex Research* 42, no. 2 (2005): 113–18; S. Sprecher, "Sexual Satisfaction in Premarital Relationships: Associations with Satisfaction, Love, Commitment, and Stability," *Journal of Sex Research* 39, no. 3 (2002): 190–96.

2 R. Rosen, D. Kountz, T. Post-Zwicker, S. Leiblum, and M. Wiegel, "Sexual Communication Skills in Residency Training: The Robert Wood Johnson Model," *Journal of Sexual Medicine* 3, no. 1 (2008): 37–46; S. T. Lindau, P. Schumm, E. O. Laumann, W. Levinson, C. A. O'Muircheartaigh, and L. J. Waite, "A Study of Sexuality and Health Among Older Adults in the United States," *New England Journal of Medicine* 357, no. 8 (2007): 762–74; M. L. Stead, L. Fallowfield, J. M. Brown, and P. Selby, "Communication about Sexual Problems and Sexual Concerns in Ovarian Cancer: Qualitative Study," *British Medical Journal* 323, no. 7317 (2007): 836–37.

3 J. Bancroft, J. Loftus, and J. S. Long, "Distress about Sex: A National Survey of Women in Heterosexual Relationships," *Archives of Sexual Behavior* 32, no. 3 (2003): 193–208; E. Haavio-Manilla and O. Kontula, "Correlates of Increased Sexual Satisfaction," *Archives of Sexual Behavior* 26, no. 4 (1997): 399–419; M. Brezsnyak and M. A. Whisman, "Sexual Desire and Relationship Functioning: The Effects of Marital Satisfaction and Power," *Journal of Sex and Marital Therapy* 30, no. 3 (2004): 119–217.

4 E. Lawrence, A. D. Rothman, R. J. Cobb, M. T. Rothman, and T. N. Bradbury, "Marital Satisfaction Across the Transition to Parenthood," *Journal of Family Psychology* 22, no. 1 (2008): 41–50; J. M. Twenge, W. K. Campbell, and C. A. Foster, "Parenthood and Marital Satisfaction: a Meta-Analytic Review," *Journal of Marriage and Family* 65, no. 3 (2003): 574–83.

5 C. Ridley, "The Ebb and Flow of Marital Lust: A Relational Approach," *The Journal of Sex Research* 43, no. 2 (2006): 144–53.

6 G. Trudel, "Sexual and Marital Life: Results of a Survey," *Journal of Sex and Marital Therapy* 28, no. 3 (2002): 229–49.

7 J. A. Hess, A. D. Fannin, and L. H. Pollom, "Creating Closeness: Discerning and Measuring Strategies for Fostering Closer Relationships," *Personal Relationships* 14, no. 3 (2007): 25–44.

8 G. Trudel, "Sexual and Marital Life: Results of a Survey," *Journal of Sex and Marital Therapy* 28, no. 3 (2002): 229–49.

9 A. Aron, C. C. Norman, E. N. Aron, C. McKenna, and R. E. Heyman, "Couples' Shared Participation in Novel and Arousing Activities," *Journal of Personality and Social Psychology* 78, no. 2 (2000): 273–84.

Resources

HEALTH INFORMATION AND REFERRALS

American College of Obstetricians and Gynecologists (ACOG)
409 12th Street, SW
PO Box 96920
Washington, DC 20090-6920
Phone: (202) 638-5577
Web: www.acog.org

International Society for the Study of Vulvovaginal Disease (ISSVD)
8814 Peppergrass Lane
Waxhaw, NC 28173
Phone: (704) 814-9493
Web: www.issvd.org
> *Patient education and referrals related to vulvar and vaginal health.*

National Vulvodynia Association (NVA)
PO Box 4491
Silver Spring, MD 20914-4491
Phone: (301) 299-0775
Web: www.nva.org
> *Information and resources for women dealing with vulvar or vaginal pain.*

The North American Menopause Society (NAMS)
PO Box 94527
Cleveland, OH 44101
Phone: (440) 442-7550
Web: www.menopause.org

COUNSELORS AND THERAPISTS

Each of the following organizations offers a way to search on their Web site so that you can identify counselors or therapists in your local area.

American Association for Marriage and Family Therapy
112 South Alfred Street
Alexandria, VA 22314-3061
Phone: (703) 838-9808
Web: www.aamft.org

American Association of Sexuality Educators, Counselors, and Therapists (AASECT)
PO Box 1960
Ashland, Virginia 23005-1960
Phone: (804) 752-0026
Web: www.aasect.org

American Psychological Association (APA)
750 First Street, NE
Washington, DC 20002-4242
Phone: (800) 374-2721
Web: www.apa.org

Society for Sex Therapy and Research
409 12th Street, SW
PO Box 96920
Washington, DC 20090-6920
Phone: (202) 863-1644
Web: www.sstarnet.org

SEXUALITY INFORMATION

Centers for Disease Control and Prevention
1600 Clifton Road
Atlanta, GA 30333
Phone: (800) CDC-INFO (800-232-4636)
Web: www.cdc.gov
> *Provides comprehensive information about sexually transmissible diseases.*

Betty Dodson with Carlin Ross
Web: www.dodsonandross.com
> *Offers comprehensive information on all aspects of women's sexuality with a Web-based community, podcasts, online store, and more.*

The Kinsey Institute for Research in Sex, Gender, and Reproduction
313 Morrison Hall
Indiana University
Bloomington, Indiana 47405
Web: www.kinseyinstitute.org
> *Information and resources related to the study of human sexuality; the Institute also houses an expansive collection of art, artifacts, and books related to human sexuality.*

Kinsey Confidential
Web: www.kinseyconfidential.org
> *As a service of the Kinsey Institute, Kinsey Confidential offers a Web-based sexuality question-and-answer service as well as audio podcasts on a variety of sexuality topics.*

Planned Parenthood Federation of America
434 West 33rd Street
New York, NY 10001
Phone: (212) 541-7800
Web: www.plannedparenthood.org
> *Provides information related to sexually transmissible diseases, family planning, contraception, and other health topics. Their Web site allows you to search for a health clinic in your local area.*

Sex Information and Education Council of Canada (SIECCAN)
850 Coxwell Ave.
Toronto, Ontario, M4C 5R1
Phone: (416) 466-5304
Web: www.sieccan.org
> *Provides resources and education related to sexuality, including research briefs and newsletters.*

Sexuality Information and Education Council of the United States (SIECUS)
1706 R Street, NW
Washington, DC 20009
Phone: (202) 265-2405
Web: www.siecus.org
> *Provides resources, fact sheets, and publications related to sexuality, including the family-friendly Families Are Talking resource for parents and their children, which can be found at www.familiesaretalking.org.*

The Body
250 West 57th Street
New York, NY 10107
Web: www.thebody.com
> *Provides resources and information related to HIV/AIDS.*

Sinclair Intimacy Institute
Web: www.bettersex.com
> *Provides DVDs and videos related to sexual enhancement and instruction.*

BOOKS
Women's Sexuality, Masturbation, and Orgasm

Barbach, Lonnie, PhD. *For Yourself: The Fulfillment of Female Sexuality.* New York: Signet, 2000.

Blank, Hanne. *Big, Big Love: A Sourcebook on Sex for People of Size and Those Who Love Them.* Oakland: Greenery Press, 2000.

Boston Women's Health Book Collective. *Nuestros Cuerpos, Nuestras Vidas.* New York: Siete Cuentos, 2003.

——. *Our Bodies, Ourselves: A New Edition for a New Era.* New York: Simon & Schuster, 2005.

Dodson, Betty. *Sex for One: The Joy of Selfloving.* New York: Three Rivers Press, 1996.

Heiman, Julia, and Joseph LoPiccolo, PhD. *Becoming Orgasmic: A Sexual and Personal Growth Program for Women.* New York: Fireside, 1987.

Hutcherson, Hilda, MD. *What Your Mother Never Told You About S-e-x.* New York: Perigree Books, 2003.

Ladas, Alice Kahn, MSS, EdD, Beverly Whipple, PhD, and John D. Perry, PhD. *The G Spot: And Other Discoveries About Human Sexuality (Revised).* New York: Holt, 2004.

Leiblum, Sandra, PhD, and Judith Sachs. *Getting the Sex You Want: A Woman's Guide to Becoming Proud, Passionate, and Pleased in Bed.* New York: Crown, 2002.

Newman, Felice. *The Whole Lesbian Sex Book: A Passionate Guide for All of Us.* San Francisco: Cleis Press, 2004.

Marriage and Relationships

Barbach, Lonnie, PhD. *For Each Other: Sharing Sexual Intimacy.* Seattle: Signet, 2001.

Easton, Dossie, and Catherine A. Liszt. *The Ethical Slut: A Guide to Infinite Sexual Possibilities.* Oakland: Greenery Press, 1997.

Gottman, John M., PhD, Julie Schwartz Gottman, PhD, and Joan DeClaire. *10 Lessons to Transform Your Marriage.* New York: Three Rivers Press, 2007.

Gottman, John M., PhD, and Joan DeClaire. *The Relationship Cure: A 5 Step Guide to Strengthening Your Marriage, Family, and Friendships.* New York: Three Rivers Press, 2002.

Gottman, John M., PhD, and Nan Silver. *The Seven Principles for Making Marriage Work.* New York: Three Rivers Press, 2000.

Hendrix, Harville, PhD. *Getting the Love You Want: A Guide for Couples* (20th anniversary edition). New York: Holt, 1998.

Perel, E. *Mating in Captivity: Unlocking Erotic Intelligence.* New York: Harper, 2007.

Schnarch, David, PhD. *Passionate Marriage: Sex, Love, and Intimacy in Emotionally Committed Relationships.* New York: Holt, 1998.

Sexual Health

Kaufman, Miriam, MD, Cory Silverberg, and Fran Odette. *The Ultimate Guide to Sex and Disability.* San Francisco: Cleis Press, 2007.

Stewart, Elizabeth G., MD, and Paula Spencer. *The V Book: A Doctor's Guide to Complete Vulvovaginal Health.* New York: Bantam, 2002.

Weiss, Marisa C., MD, and Ellen Weiss. *Living Beyond Breast Cancer: A Survivor's Guide for When Treatment Ends and the Rest of Your Life Begins.* New York: Three Rivers Press, 1998.

Pregnancy and Birth

The Boston Women's Health Book Collective. *Our Bodies, Ourselves: Pregnancy and Birth.* New York: Touchstone, 2008.

Westheimer, Dr. Ruth K., and Amos Grünebaum, MD, FACOG. *Dr. Ruth's Pregnancy Guide for Couples.* New York: Routledge, 1999.

Menopause and Aging

The Boston Women's Health Book Collective. *Our Bodies, Ourselves: Menopause.* New York: Touchstone, 2006.

Levine, Suzanne Braun. *Inventing the Rest of Our Lives: Women in Second Adulthood.* New York: Viking, 2004.

Northrup, Christiane, MD. *The Wisdom of Menopause (2nd Edition).* New York: Bantam, 2006.

Price, Joan. *Better Than I Ever Expected: Straight Talk About Sex After Sixty.* Emeryville: Seal Press, 2005.

Schwartz, Dr. Pepper. *Prime: Adventures and Advice on Sex, Love, and the Sensual Years.* New York: Collins Living, 2008.

Sexual Enhancement and Instruction Guides

Blue, Violet. *The Ultimate Guide to Fellatio: How to Go Down on a Man and Give Him Mind-Blowing Pleasure.* San Francisco: Cleis Press, 2002.

Brisben, Patty. *Pure Romance Between the Sheets: Find Your Best Sexual Self and Enhance Your Intimate Relationship.* New York: Atria, 2008.

Inkeles, Gordon. *The Art of Sensual Massage.* Bayside: Arcata Arts, 2000.

Kerner, Ian. *She Comes First: The Thinking Man's Guide to Pleasuring a Woman.* New York: ReganBooks, 2004.

Morin, Jack, PhD. *Anal Pleasure and Health: A Guide for Men and Women.* San Francisco: Down There Press, 1998.

Paget, Lou. *The Great Lover Playbook: 365 Sexual Tips and Techniques to Keep the Fires Burning All Year Long.* New York: Gotham Books, 2005.

Sundahl, Deborah. *Female Ejaculation and the G-Spot.* Alameda: Hunter House, 2003.

Taormino, Tristan. *The Ultimate Guide to Anal Sex for Women, 2nd Edition.* San Francisco: Cleis Press, 2006.

Venning, Rachel, and Claire Cavanah. *Sex Toys 101: A Playfully Uninhibited Guide.* New York: Fireside, 2003.

Winks, Cathy, and Anne Semans. *The New Good Vibrations Guide to Sex.* San Francisco: Cleis Press, 2002.

Women's Erotica

Barbach, Lonnie, PhD. *The Erotic Edge: 22 Erotic Stories for Couples*. New York: Plume, 1996.

Blue, Violet. *Best Women's Erotica 2009*. San Francisco: Cleis Press, 2008.

Friday, Nancy. *My Secret Garden: Women's Sexual Fantasies*. New York: Pocket Books, 2008.

Jameson, Jenna, and OliverSmith, M. Catherine. *Something Blue: Jenna Tales*. Savannah: Sounds Publishing, 2008.

Semans, Anne, and Cathy Winks. *Sex Toy Tales*. San Francisco: Down There Press, 1998.

Abuse, Assault, and Trauma

Bass, Ellen, and Louise Thornton, editors. *I Never Told Anyone: Writings by Women Survivors of Child Sexual Abuse*. New York: Harper Perennial, 1983.

Bass, Ellen, and Laura Davis. *The Courage to Heal: A Guide for Women Survivors of Child Sexual Abuse*. New York: Harper Perennial, 1994.

Dugan, Megan Kennedy, and Roger R. Hock. *It's My Life Now: Starting Over After an Abusive Relationship or Domestic Violence*. New York: Routeledge, 2006.

Male Sexuality

Metz, Michael E., PhD, and Barry W. McCarthy, PhD. *Coping with Erectile Dysfunction: How to Regain Confidence and Enjoy Great Sex*. Oakland: New Harbinger Publications, 2004.

———. *Coping with Premature Ejaculation: How to Overcome PE, Please Your Partner, and Have Great Sex*. Oakland: New Harbinger Publications, 2004.

Milsten, Richard, MD, and Julian Slowinski, PsyD. *The Sexual Male: Problems and Solutions*. New York: W.W. Norton & Company, 2000.

Zilbergeld, Bernie, PhD. *The New Male Sexuality*. New York: Bantam, 1999.

Parenting

Haffner, Debra W. *Beyond the Big Talk: Every Parent's Guide to Raising Sexually Healthy Teens, Second Edition*. New York: Newmarket Press, 2008.

———. *From Diapers to Dating: A Parent's Guide to Raising Sexually Healthy Children from Infancy to Middle School*. New York: Newmarket Press, 2004.

Harris, Robie H. *It's Not the Stork: A Book About Girls, Boys, Babies, Bodies, Families, and Friends*. Cambridge: Candlewick, 2008.

Kerner, I., and H. Raykeil. *Love in the Time of Colic: The New Parents' Guide to Getting It On Again*. New York: Collins Living, 2009.

Mindfulness

Hanh, Thich Nhat. *The Miracle of Mindfulness*. Boston: Beacon Press, 1999.

Kabat-Zinn, Jon. *Mindfulness for Beginners*. Louisville, CO: Sounds True, Inc, 2006. (Audio CD).

IN-HOME SEX TOY PARTY COMPANIES

In-home parties are independently run by women throughout the world. Visit their Web sites to find a party facilitator near you.

Ann Summers (UK)
www.annsummers.com

Passion Parties (US)
www.passionparties.com

Pleasure Box (Australia/New Zealand)
www.pleasurebox.com.au

Pure Romance (US)
www.pureromance.com

WOMAN-FRIENDLY ONLINE SEX TOY SHOPS AND BOUTIQUES

A Woman's Touch
www.a-womans-touch.com

Babeland
www.babeland.com

Blowfish
www.blowfish.com

Come As You Are
www.comeasyouare.com

Early to Bed
www.early2bed.com

G Boutique
www.boutiqueg.com

Good Vibrations
www.goodvibes.com

MyPleasure
www.mypleasure.com

Myla
www.myla.com

S3 Safe Sex Store
www.s3safesexstore.com

The Pleasure Chest
www.thepleasurechest.com

Tulip
www.mytulip.com

Acknowledgments

All books are borne of the time, talents, and expertise of numerous individuals. I am grateful, first and foremost, to the many students I have taught in human sexuality classes at Indiana University, as well as to the women and men who have reached out to me for help with their sex lives. I feel touched by the trust that so many people have shown by sharing their very personal feelings and concerns with me.

I am also grateful to my agent, Kate Lee, who understood the need for a book centered on pleasure and trusted in my abilities to translate scientific information about sex into practical yet fun suggestions that individuals can use to improve their sexual lives. I would like to thank Leigh Haber for her enthusiastic support of my ideas and my editor, Julie Will, for gracefully helping to clarify my words in ways that stayed true to these ideas and to the science behind them. In addition, I am indebted to Beth Tarson for her innovative efforts related to sharing the "feel good" message and to Larissa Silva for her patience and kindness.

I feel fortunate to work with smart, engaging, and warm-hearted colleagues at the Center for Sexual Health Promotion and the Kinsey Institute for Research in Sex, Gender and Reproduction at Indiana University, all of whom have shaped my thinking about sexuality and supported my passion for educating others about sex. In particular, I would like to acknowledge and thank Jennifer Bass, John Bancroft, Brian Dodge, Dennis Fortenberry, Bob Goodman, Cynthia Graham, Catherine Johnson, Julia Heiman, Carol McCord, Michael Reece, June Reinisch, Meredith Reynolds, Stephanie Sanders, and Mohammad Torabi.

I am also grateful to my present and past editors at *Men's Health, Time Out Chicago,* and *Velocity,* all of whom have valued the importance of making accurate, science-based information about sex available to the women and men who are curious about it. Thank you to Matt Bean, Amy Carr, Jim Lenahan, Tom Nord, Chad Schlegel, Frank Sennett, Ruth Welte, and Cecilia Wong. In addition, I am thankful to have been encouraged at various stages of my life by Chris Ashford, Patty Brisben, Peter Greer, Ian Kerner, Erin Hoschouer Lapham, Reggie McKnight, Christine Robinson, and Russell Weatherspoon.

Heartfelt thanks go to my friends and family (especially Ariane, Dave, Erica, Jessica, Nancy, Susie, Gammy, Jimmy, and Roberta) who gave me the time, space, and encouragement to focus on writing this book. I am appreciative of Steve for letting me turn his home into my office and to the staff of Food Matters in Alexandria, Virginia, where several chapters of this book were written over lingering lunches. Also, I am grateful to James for his patience, support, feedback, and willingness to have a number of our meals interrupted by book-related discussions. My sister, Laura, read through early versions of chapters and gave me helpful feedback, for which I am indebted to her. Finally, I am thankful to my parents and grandparents who raised me with a love of books, education, and the simple.

Index

Boldface page references indicate illustrations. Underscored references indicate boxed text.

•

●

●

●